Practical Record Book of

Nursing Foundations

for BSc Nursing Students

As per the Revised INC Syllabus (2021-22) for BSc Nursing

Nursing Knowledge Tree
An Initiative by CBS Nursing Division

Practical Record Book of

Nursing Foundations

for BSc Nursing Students

As per the Revised INC Syllabus (2021-22) for BSc Nursing

Ravindra HN PhD (N), MPhil, MSc (N), BAMS (AM), MA (Sociology)
Dean
Faculty of Nursing
Parul University, Vadodara, Gujarat

CBSPD
Dedicated to Education

CBS Publishers & Distributors Pvt Ltd

• New Delhi • Bengaluru • Chennai • Kochi • Kolkata • Lucknow • Mumbai
• Hyderabad • Jharkhand • Nagpur • Patna • Pune • Uttarakhand

Practical Record Book of

Nursing Foundations

for BSc Nursing Students

ISBN: 978-93-90619-60-3

Reprint: 2026, 2024

First Edition: 2022

Published by **Satish Kumar Jain** and produced by **Varun Jain** for

CBS Publishers & Distributors Pvt Ltd

4819/XI Prahlad Street, 24 Ansari Road, Daryaganj, New Delhi 110 002, India.

Ph: +91-11-23289259, 23266861, 23266867 Website: www.cbspd.com

Fax: 011-23243014

e-mail: delhi@cbspd.com; cbspubs@airtelmail.in.

Corporate Office: 204 FIE, Industrial Area, Patparganj, Delhi 110 092

Ph: +91-11-4934 4934 Fax: 4934 4935

e-mail: feedback@cbspd.com

Branches

- **Bengaluru:** Seema House 2975, 17th Cross, K.R. Road, Banashankari 2nd Stage, Bengaluru 560 070, Karnataka
  Ph: +91-80-26771678/79 Fax: +91-80-26771680 e-mail: bangalore@cbspd.com
- **Chennai:** 7, Subbaraya Street, Shenoy Nagar, Chennai 600 030, Tamil Nadu
  Ph: +91-44-26680620, 26681266 Fax: +91-44-42032115 e-mail: chennai@cbspd.com
- **Kochi:** 68/1534, 35, 36-Power House Road, Opp. KSEB, Cochin-682018, Kochi, Kerala
  Ph: +91-484-4059061-65 Fax: +91-484-4059065 e-mail: kochi@cbspd.com
- **Kolkata:** Hind Ceramics Compound, 1st Floor, 147, Nilganj Road, Belghoria, Kolkata-700056, West Bengal
  Ph: +91-033-2563-3055/56 e-mail: kolkata@cbspd.com
- **Lucknow:** Basement, Khushnuma Complex, 7-Meerabai Marg (Behind Jawahar Bhawan), Lucknow-226001, Uttar Pradesh
  Ph: +0522-4000032 e-mail: tiwari.lucknow@cbspd.com
- **Mumbai:** PWD Shed, Gala No. 25/26, Ramchandra Bhatt Marg, Next to J.J. Hospital Gate No. 2, Opp. Union Bank of India, Noor Baug, Mumbai-400009, Maharashtra
  Ph: +91-22-66661880/89 Fax: +91-22-24902342 e-mail: mumbai@cbspd.com

Representatives

- **Hyderabad** +91-9885175004
- **Nagpur** +91-9421945513
- **Pune** +91-9623451994
- **Jharkhand** +91-9811541605
- **Patna** +91-9334159340
- **Uttarakhand** +91-9716462459

Printed at: Rashtriya Printers Delhi-110095

CBS Nursing Knowledge Tree

Extends its Tribute to

Florence Nightingale

For glorifying the role of women as nurses,
For holding the title of " The Lady with the Lamp,"
For working tirelessly for humanity—
Florence Nightingale will always be
remembered for her
selfless and memorable services to the
human race.

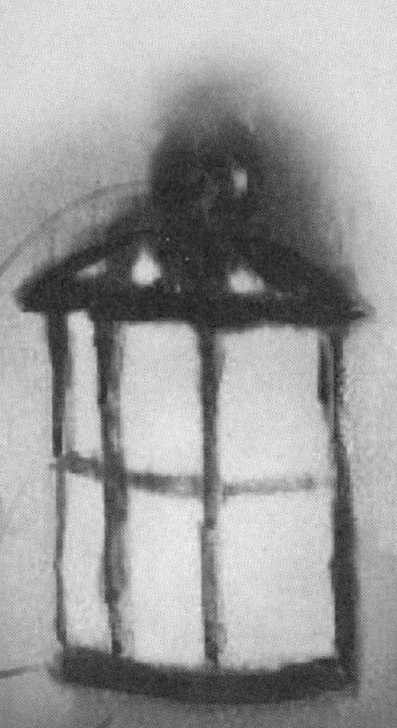

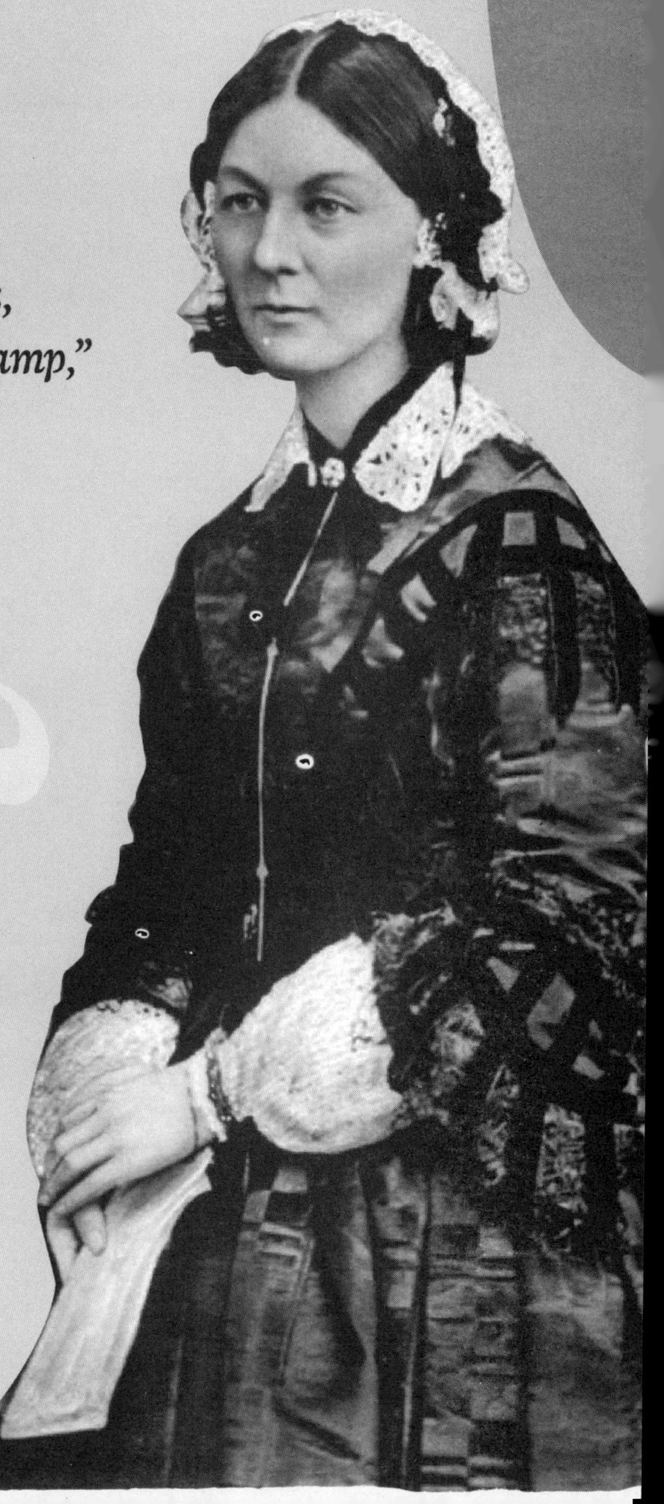

Florence Nightingale
(May 1820 – August 1910)

Dedicated to

All Nursing Students

Preface

It gives me immense pleasure to introduce the practical record book for the nursing foundation as per the revised BSc nursing guidelines program laid down by Indian Nursing Council 2020. Nursing is a highly skilled and renowned profession. It always produces knowledgeable competent nurses and midwives with clear critical thinking skills who are caring, motivated, assertive, and well-disciplined responding to the changing needs of the profession, health care delivery system, and society.

Nursing professionals and students are challenged to assume multidimensional responsibilities for providing the best nursing services under various health care settings. Therefore, as per curriculum regulations, all nursing students are imposed to uphold theoretical and practical skills, while pursuing the BSc nursing degree.

This practical record book is organized as per the requirement of nursing foundation subject for first-year BSc nursing students following the revised BSc nursing program laid down by Indian Nursing Council 2020.

Newly included, fall risk assessment, pressure sore assessment, practical proforma, and guidelines are added in this practical record book to provide broad knowledge and guidance to students, which will help students to provide need-based care to the clients and complete their practical requirements in the first year BSc nursing successfully.

I hope that this practical record book will be helpful to build student's critical thinking skills and comprehensive knowledge while delivering the client's care and completing the practical requirements.

I sincerely welcome the feedback from the readers, and beneficiaries of this practical book that would enrich my knowledge and good suggestions will be incorporated in the next edition.

Ravindra HN

Reviewers

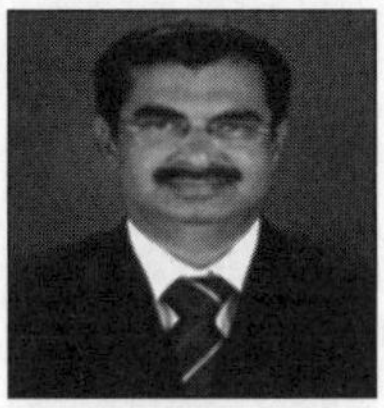

BA Yathikumara Swamy Gowda
Principal
Alva's College of Nursing
Moodbidri, Dakshina Kannada
Karnataka

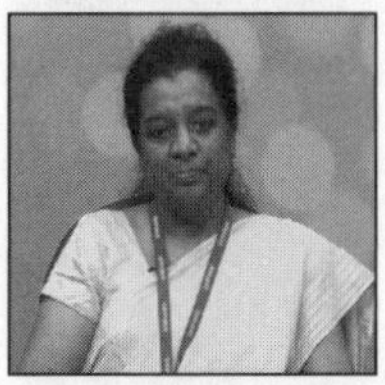

BV Kathyayani
Professor cum Principal
NIMHANS College of Nursing Bangalore
Karnataka

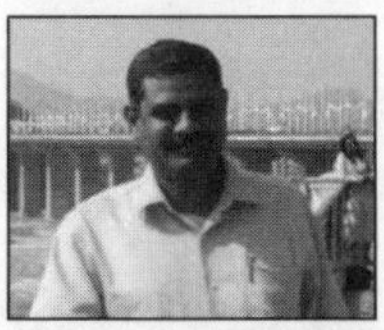

Chandra Shekhar
Professor and Principal
Adichunchanagiri College of Nursing
Mandya, Karnataka

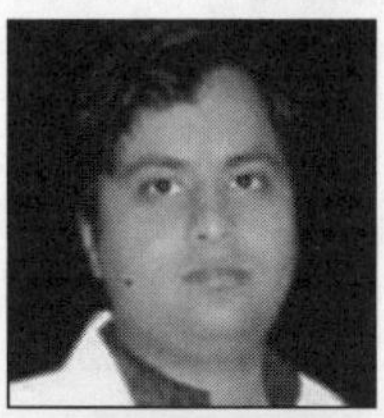

Devendra Varma
Himalaya Institute of Higher Education
Patna, Bihar

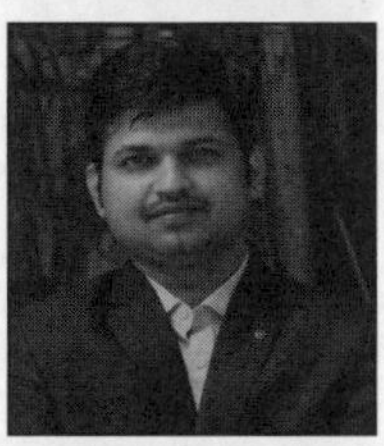

Devraj Singh Chouhan
Associate Professor and Head
Mental Health Nursing Department
Parul Institute of Nursing
Parul University
Vadodara, Gujarat

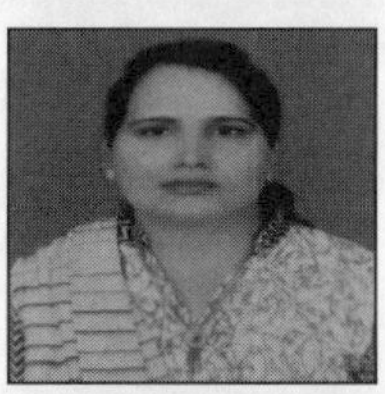

Indravathi Pandey
Principal
Government College of Nursing
Surat, Gujarat

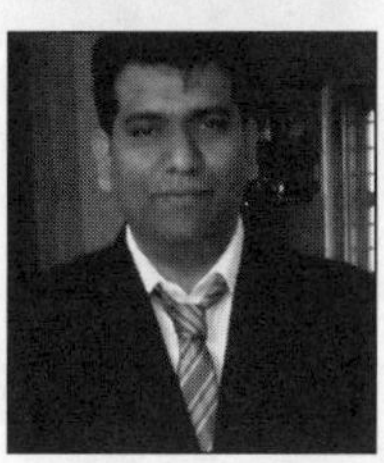

Jayesh Patidar
Professor and Vice Principal
Joitiba College of Nursing
Bhandu, Gujarat

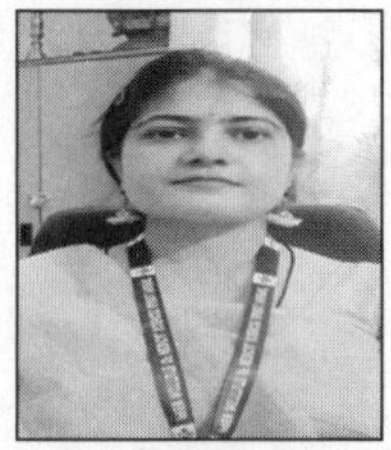

Nidhi Sharma
Professor cum Vice Principal
Prem Institute of Medical Sciences
Baroli, Panipat, Haryana

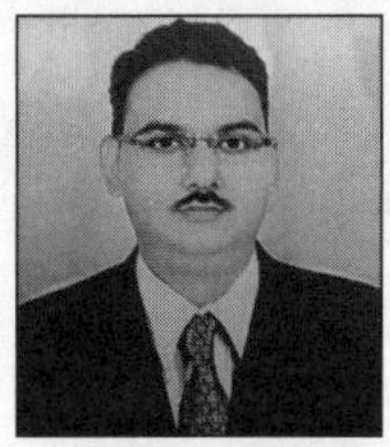

Pavan Kumar Jain
Lecturer
Government School of Nursing
Udaipur, Rajasthan

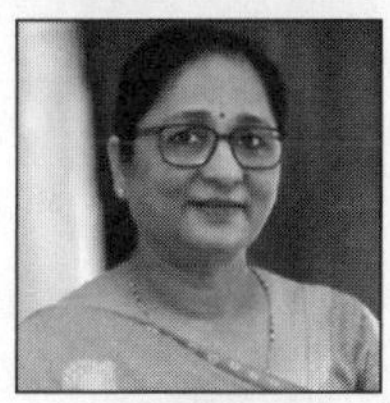

Prabha K Dasila
Professor and Director
Mahatma Gandhi Mission
Institute of Health Sciences
College of Nursing
Navi Mumbai, Maharashtra

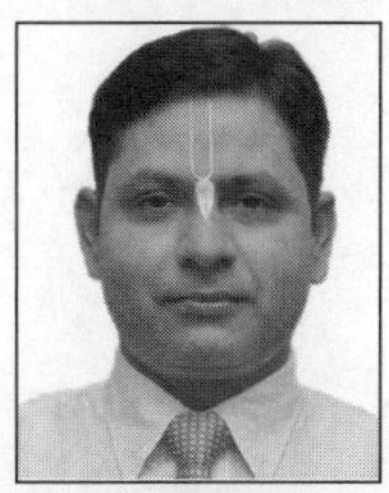

Rajesh Kumar Sharma
Associate Professor and Head
Critical Care Nursing Department
Himalayan College of Nursing
Swami Rama Himalayan University
Dehradun, Uttarakhand

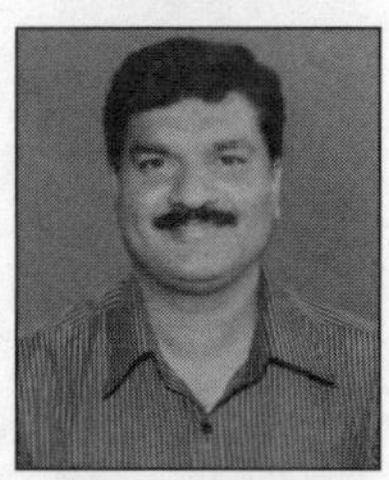

Ravish Kumar
Professor
Government College of Nursing
Hubli, Karnataka

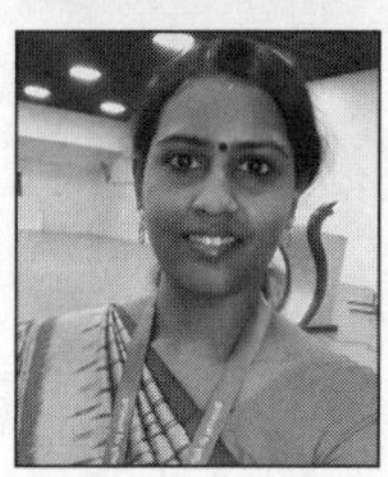

Rose Mary George
Professor and Head
Medical-Surgical Nursing Department
Parul Institute of Nursing
Parul University
Vadodara, Gujarat

The names of the reviewers are arranged in alphabetical order.

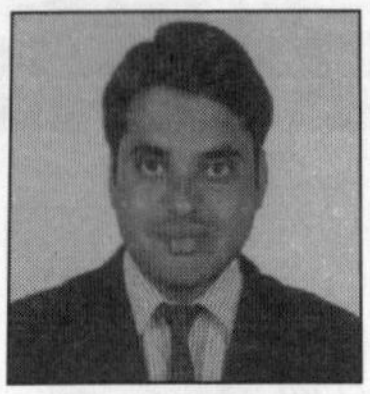

Sanjay Shinde
Professor and Head
Child Health Nursing Department
Parul Institute of Nursing
Parul University
Vadodara, Gujarat

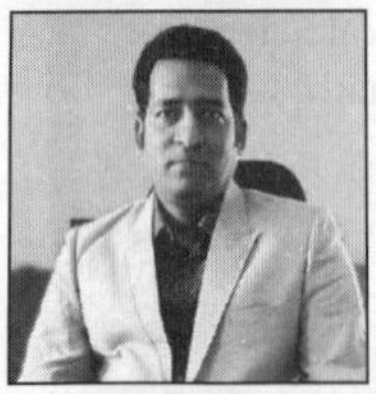

Sathish Biradar
Principal
School of Nursing
PP Savani University
Surat, Gujarat

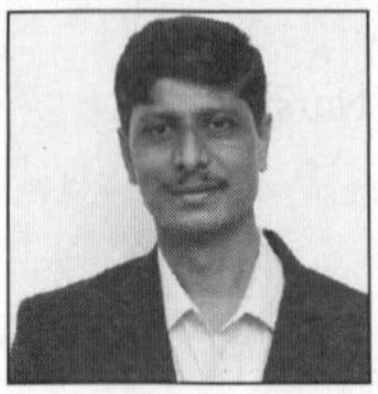

Siddaram Sarathe
Professor
Manikaka Topawala Institute of Nursing
Charusat University
Anand, Gujarat

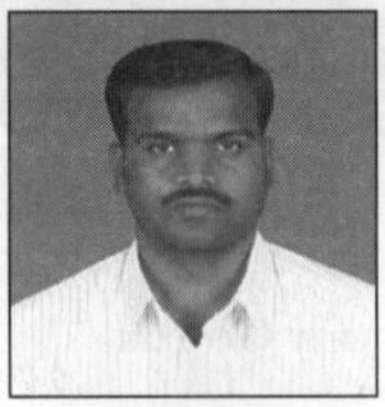

T Sivabalan
Professor and Principal
Pravara Institute of Medical Sciences
Deemed University
College of Nursing
Loni (BK), Maharashtra

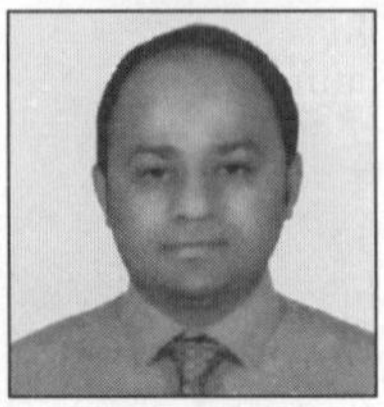

Vimlesh Vyas (PhD Scholar)
Associate Professor
Patidar Nursing Institute
Ujjain, Madhya Pradesh

The names of the reviewers are arranged in alphabetical order.

Syllabus

NURSING FOUNDATION

Theory: 6 Credits (120 hours)

Sl. no.	Course content	Time (Hours)
1.	**Introduction to Health and Illness** • Concept of health—definitions (WHO), dimensions • Maslow's hierarchy of needs • Health-illness continuum • Factors influencing health • Causes and risk factors for developing illnesses • Illness—types, illness behavior, impact of illness on patient and family	5 (T)
2.	**Health Care Delivery Systems—Introduction of Basic Concepts and Meanings** • Levels of illness prevention—primary (health promotion), secondary and tertiary • Levels of care—primary, secondary, and tertiary • Types of health care agencies/services—hospitals, clinics, hospice, rehabilitation centers, extended care facilities • Hospitals—types, organization, and functions • Health care teams in hospitals—members and their role	5 (T)
3.	**History of Nursing and Nursing as a Profession** • History of nursing, history of nursing in India • Contributions of Florence Nightingale • Nursing—definition—nurse, nursing, concepts, philosophy, objectives, characteristics, nature, and scope of nursing/nursing practice, functions of nurse, qualities of a nurse, categories of nursing personnel • Nursing as a profession—definition and characteristics/criteria of a profession • Values—introduction—meaning and importance • Code of ethics and professional conduct for nurses—introduction	12 (T)
4.	**Communication a Nurse-Patient Relationship** • Communication—levels, elements and process, types, modes, factors influencing communication • Methods of effective communication/therapeutic communication techniques • Barriers to effective communication/nontherapeutic communication techniques • Professional communication • Helping relationships (nurse-patient relationship)—purposes and phases • Communicating effectively with patients, families and team members • Maintaining effective human relations and communication with vulnerable groups (children, women, physically and mentally challenged and elderly)	8 (T) 3 (SL)
5.	**Documentation and Reporting** • Documentation—purposes of reports and records • Confidentiality • Types of client records/common recordkeeping forms • Methods/systems of documentation/recording guidelines for documentation • Do's and don'ts of documentation/legal guidelines for documentation/recording • Reporting—change of shift reports, transfer reports, incident reports	4 (T) 2 (SL)

Contd...

<table>
<tr><th>Sl. no.</th><th>Course content</th><th>Time (Hours)</th></tr>
<tr><td>6.</td><td>Vital Signs
• Guidelines for taking vital signs
• Body temperature:
▪ Definition, physiology, regulation, factors affecting body temperature
▪ Assessment of body temperature—sites, equipment, and technique
▪ Temperature alterations—hyperthermia, heat cramps, heat exhaustion, heatstroke, hypothermia
▪ Fever/pyrexia—definition, causes, stages, types
• Nursing management
▪ Hot and cold applications
• Pulse:
▪ Definition, physiology, and regulation, characteristics, factors affecting pulse
▪ Assessment of pulse—sites, equipment, and technique
▪ Alterations in pulse
• Respiration:
▪ Definition, physiology and regulation, mechanics of breathing, characteristics, factors affecting respiration
▪ Assessment of respiration—a technique
▪ Arterial oxygen saturation
▪ Alterations in respiration
• Blood pressure:
▪ Definition, physiology and regulation, characteristics, factors affecting BP
▪ Assessment of BP—sites, equipment and technique, common errors in BP assessment
▪ Alterations in blood pressure
• Documenting vital signs</td><td>15 (T)
20 (SL)</td></tr>
<tr><td>7.</td><td>Equipment and Linen
• Types—disposables and reusable
▪ Linen, rubber goods, glassware, metal, plastics, furniture
• Introduction—indent, maintenance, inventory</td><td>3 (T)</td></tr>
<tr><td>8.</td><td>Introduction to Infection Control in Clinical Setting Infection
• Nature of infection
• Chain of infection
• Types of infection
• Stages of infection
• Factors increasing susceptibility to infection
• Body defense against infection—inflammatory response and immune response
• Health care-associated infection (nosocomial infection)
Introductory Concept of Asepsis—
Medical and Surgical Asepsis
Precautions
• Hand hygiene
• Hand washing and use of hand rub
• Use of personal protective equipment (PPE)
• Standard precautions
Biomedical Waste Management
• Types of hospital waste, waste segregation and hazards—introduction</td><td>10 (T)
3 (SL)</td></tr>
</table>

Contd...

Sl. no.	Course content	Time (Hours)
9.	**Comfort, Rest and Sleep and Pain** • Comfort ▪ Factors influencing comfort ▪ Types of beds including latest beds, purposes of bed-making ▪ Therapeutic positions ▪ Comfort devices • Sleep and rest ▪ Physiology of sleep ▪ Factors affecting sleep ▪ Promoting rest and sleep ▪ Sleep disorders • Pain (discomfort) ▪ Physiology ▪ Common cause of pain ▪ Types ▪ Assessment—pain scales and narcotic scales. Pharmacological and nonpharmacological pain-relieving measures—use of narcotics, TENS devices, PCA ▪ Invasive techniques of pain management ▪ Any other newer measures ▪ Complementary and alternative healing modalities (CAM)	**15 (T)** **15 (SL)**
10.	**Promoting Safety in Health Care Environment** • Physical environment—temperature, humidity, noise, ventilation, light, odor, pest control • Reduction of physical hazards—fire, accidents • Fall risk assessment • Role of nurse in providing safe and clean environment • Safety devices ▪ Restraints—types, purposes, indications, legal implications and consent, application of restraints, skill and practice guidelines ▪ Other safety devices—side rails, grab bars, ambu alarms, non-skid slippers, etc.	**5 (T)** **3 (SL)**
11.	**Hospital Admission and Discharge** • Admission to the hospital unit and preparation of unit ▪ Admission bed ▪ Admission procedure ▪ Medico-legal issues ▪ Roles and responsibilities of the nurse • Discharge from the hospital ▪ Types—planned discharge, LAMA and, abscond, referrals and transfers ▪ Discharge planning ▪ Discharge procedure ▪ Medico-legal issues ▪ Roles and responsibilities of the nurse ▪ Care of the unit after discharge	**6 (T)** **2 (SL)**

Contd...

Sl. no.	Course content	Time (Hours)
12.	**Mobility and Immobility** • Elements of normal movement, alignment and posture, joint mobility, balance, coordinated movement principles of body mechanics • Factors affecting body alignment and activity • Exercise—types and benefits • Effects of Immobility • Maintenance of normal body alignment and activity • Alteration in body alignment and mobility • Nursing interventions for impaired body alignment and mobility—assessment, types, devices used, method ▪ Range of motion exercises ▪ Muscle-strengthening exercises ▪ Maintaining body alignment—positions ▪ Moving, lifting, or transferring ▪ Walking, assisting clients with ambulation • Care of patients with immobility using nursing process approach • Care of patients with casts and splints	**8 (T)** **10 (SL)**
13.	**Patient Education** • Patient teaching—importance, purposes, process • Integrating nursing process in patient teaching	**4 (T)** **2 (SL)**
14.	**First Aid*** • Definition, basic principles, scope and rules • First aid management ▪ Wounds, hemorrhage and shock ▪ Musculoskeletal injuries—fractures, dislocation, muscle injuries ▪ Transportation of injured persons ▪ Respiratory emergencies and basic CPR ▪ Unconsciousness ▪ Foreign bodies—skin, eye, ear, nose, throat and stomach ▪ Burns and scalds ▪ Poisoning, bites and stings ▪ Frostbite and effects of heat ▪ Community emergencies	**20 (T)** **20 (SL)**

PRACTICAL

Placement: I & II Semester

Clinical Practicum: 2 Credits (160 hours)

10 weeks × 16 hours per week

General objectives: Students will be able to apply the nursing process and perform the various procedures through comprehensive nursing care to ill clients.

Specific objectives: After completion of the Clinical Practicum of I & II Semester BSc Nursing program, the students will be able to:

- Maintain effective human relations (projecting professional image).
- Communicate effectively with patient, families and team members.
- Demonstrate skills in techniques of recording and reporting.
- Demonstrate skill in monitoring vital signs.
- Care for patients with altered vital signs.
- Demonstrate skill in implementing standard precautions and use of PPE.
- Demonstrate skill in meeting the comfort needs of the patients.
- Provide a safe and clean environment.
- Demonstrate skill in admission, transfer, and discharge of a patient.
- Demonstrate skill in caring for patients with restricted mobility.
- Plan and provide appropriate health teaching following the principles.
- Acquire skills in assessing and performing First Aid during emergencies.

Clinical unit	Duration (in weeks)	Learning outcomes	Procedural competencies/ clinical skills (supervised clinical practice)	Clinical requirements	Assessment methods
General medical/ surgical wards	2 (two weeks)	• Maintain effective human relations (projecting professional image) • Communicate effectively with patient, families and team members • Demonstrate skills in techniques of recording and reporting	**Communication and Nurse-patient Relationship:** • Maintaining communication with patient and family and interpersonal relationship • Documentation and reporting ▪ Documenting patient care and procedures ▪ Verbal report ▪ Written report		• OSCE

Contd...

Clinical unit	Duration (in weeks)	Learning outcomes	Procedural competencies/ clinical skills (supervised clinical practice)	Clinical requirements	Assessment methods
	2	• Demonstrate skill in monitoring vital signs • Care for patients with altered vital signs • Demonstrate skill in implementing standard precautions and use of PPE	**Vital Signs:** • Monitor/measure and document vital signs in a graphic sheet ▪ Temperature (oral, tympanic, axillary) ▪ Pulse (apical and peripheral pulses) ▪ Respiration ▪ Blood pressure ▪ Pulse oximetry • Interpret and report alteration • Cold applications—cold compress, ice cold, sponging • Care of equipment—thermometer, BP apparatus, stethoscope, pulse oximeter **Infection Control in Clinical Settings:** • Hand hygiene • Use of PPE	Care of patients with alterations in vital signs—1	• Assessment of clinical skills using checklist • OSCE
	3	Demonstrate skill in meeting the comfort needs of the patients	**Comfort, Rest and Sleep, Pain and Promoting Safety in Health Care Environment: Comfort, Rest and Sleep:** • Bed making: ▪ Open ▪ Closed ▪ Occupied ▪ Postoperative or cardiac bed ▪ Fracture bed • Comfort devices: ▪ Over bed table/ cardiac table ▪ Pillow ▪ Back rest ▪ Bed cradle		• Assessment of clinical skills using checklist • OSCE

Contd...

Clinical unit	Duration (in weeks)	Learning outcomes	Procedural competencies/ clinical skills (supervised clinical practice)	Clinical requirements	Assessment methods
		Provide safe and clean environment	• Therapeutic positions: ▪ Fowler's (low, semi, high) ▪ Supine ▪ Lateral ▪ Prone ▪ Sims' ▪ Trendelenburg ▪ Dorsal recumbent ▪ Lithotomy ▪ Knee chest **Pain:** • Pain assessment and provision for comfort **Promoting Safety in Health Care Environment:** • Care of patient's unit • Use of safety devices • Side rails • Restraints (physical) • Fall risk assessment and post fall assessment		
	2	Demonstrate skill in admission, transfer, and discharge of a patient	**Hospital Admission and Discharge, Mobility and Immobility and Patient Education:** Hospital admission and discharge proforma and document: • Admission • Transfer • Planned Discharge		• Assessment of clinical skills using checklist • OSCE
		• Demonstrate skill in caring for patients with restricted mobility • Plan and provide appropriate health teaching following the principles	**Mobility and Immobility:** • Range of motion exercises • Assist patient in: ▪ Moving ▪ Turning ▪ Logrolling • Changing position of helpless patient • Transferring (bed to and from chair/wheelchair/ stretcher) *patient education*		

Contd...

Clinical unit	Duration (in weeks)	Learning outcomes	Procedural competencies/ clinical skills (supervised clinical practice)	Clinical requirements	Assessment methods
	1	Demonstrate skills in assessing and performing first aid during emergencies	**First Aid and Emergencies:** • Bandaging techniques **Basic bandages:** • Circular • Spiral • Reverse-spiral • Recurrent • Figure of eight **Special bandages:** • Caplin • Eye/ear bandage • Jaw bandage • Shoulder spica • Thumb spica • Triangular bandage/ sling (head and limbs) • Binders	• Module completion • National Disaster Management Authority (NDMA) • First Aid module (to complete it in clinical if not completed during lab)	• Assessment of clinical skills using checklist • OSCE (first aid competencies)

Contents

Student's Identification Profile

Paste Your Passport Size Photograph

Name of the Student: ______________________

Registration No./Enrolment No.: ______________________

College Roll No.: ______________________

Course/Batch Year: ______________________

Subject: ______________________

Batch: ______________________

Name of the Institute/College: ______________________

Address of the Institute/College: ______________________

: ______________________

: ______________________

: ______________________

Signature of the Student	Signature of the Subject Coordinator	Signature of the Principal

COURSE OF INSTRUCTION

Course/subject title	Total credits	Total hours (theory skill lab, clinical)
Communicative English	2	40
Applied Anatomy and Applied Physiology	3	60 + 60
Applied Sociology and Applied Psychology	3	60 + 60
Nursing Foundation-I including First Aid Module—Theory	6	120
Nursing Foundation-I including First Aid Module—Practical	04	240 (Skill lab–80, Clinical–160)
Self-study	–	40
Co-curricular	–	40
Total	**24**	**720**

SCHEME OF EXAMINATION

Course	Assessment (marks)				
	Internal	End semester college exam	End semester university exam	Hours	Total marks
Theory					
Communicative English	25	25	–	2	50
Applied Anatomy and Applied Physiology	25	–	75	3	100
Applied Sociology and Applied Psychology	25	–	75	3	100
Nursing Foundations-I	*25	–	–	–	–
Practical					
Nursing Foundations-I	*25	–	–	–	–

***Will be added to the internal marks of Nursing Foundation-II Theory and Practical respectively in the next semester (Total weightage remains the same)**

Semester I

LIST OF PRACTICAL REQUIREMENTS

Sl. no.	Name of clinical requirement	Maximum marks	Marks obtained	Signature of the Teacher
I.	**History Taking (2)**			
	1.			
	2.			
II.	**Physical Examination (2)**			
	1.			
	2.			
III.	**Fall Risk Assessment (2)**			
	1.			
	2.			
IV.	**Pressure Sore Assessment (2)**			
	1.			
	2.			
V.	**Nursing Process (2)**			
	1.			
	2.			
VI.	**Completion of First Aid Module**			
VII.	**Completion of Health Assessment Module**			

HISTORY TAKING–1 (MEDICAL)

BIOGRAPHICAL DATA OF PATIENT

Name of the Patient: ______________________ Age: ________ Gender: ____________

Date of Health History Collection: ______________________ Date of Admission: ____________

Hospital/IP No: ______________________ Language Spoken: ______________________

Marital Status: ____________ Educational Status: ____________ Religion: ____________

Occupation: ______________________ Provisional Diagnosis: ______________________

Treatment under Doctor: ____

Name of the procedure (if surgery/procedure done): ______________________________

CHIEF COMPLAINTS

____

____

____

____

____

HISTORY OF PRESENT ILLNESS

____

____

____

____

____

PAST MEDICAL HISTORY

- Past illness and treatment (birth problem/childhood illness/immunization history): History of blood transfusion:
- Any allergic history (food/medication/other):
- Any other relevant (physical/psychological or mental illness):
- Previous hospitalization:

SOCIOECONOMIC STATUS

FAMILY HISTORY OF ANY ILLNESS

Family Tree Diagram:

Genogram Key	
Female	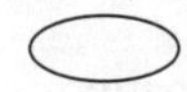
Male	
Patient	
Deceased	 OR 
Cause of death	( )
Adoption (vertical)	| ====
Consanguinity	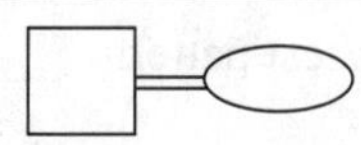

(For reference)

History of chronic illness such as: (diabetes mellitus, hypertension, coronary artery disease, renal disease, psychiatric illness, cancer, etc.): ____

____

____

History of any recent death in the family: ____

____

____

History of any hereditary disease or communicable disease in the family: ____

____

PERSONAL HISTORY

- Personal hygiene: ____

  ____

- Dietary history (veg/non-veg/meal pattern, any practice): ______________________
____
- Elimination pattern: ______________________
____
- Physical activities and exercises: ______________________
____
- Work pattern (type, level of job satisfaction, work stress, etc.): ______________________
____
- Sleeping/rest pattern: ______________________
____
- Hobbies: ______________________
____
- Use of any addictive substances: ______________________
____
- Relationship with patient, friends, significant others: ______________________
____
- Social activities and religious activities: ______________________
____

PHYSICAL EXAMINATION

GENERAL APPEARANCE

- **Level of consciousness**: (consciousness/unconsciousness/semi-consciousness/coma/confused, etc.): ______________________________
- Orientation (time/place/person): ______________________________
- Mood: ______________________________
- Activity: ______________________________
- Body built: ______________________________

Weight: ____________ **Height** (inches/cm): ____________ **BMI** (weight (kg)/height in meter^2): ____________

VITAL SIGNS

Day/Date	Temperature (In °F/°C)	Pulse (beats/min)	Respiration (breaths/min)	Blood pressure (mm Hg)	Pain score on VAS

VISUAL ANALOGUE PAIN (VAS) SCALE

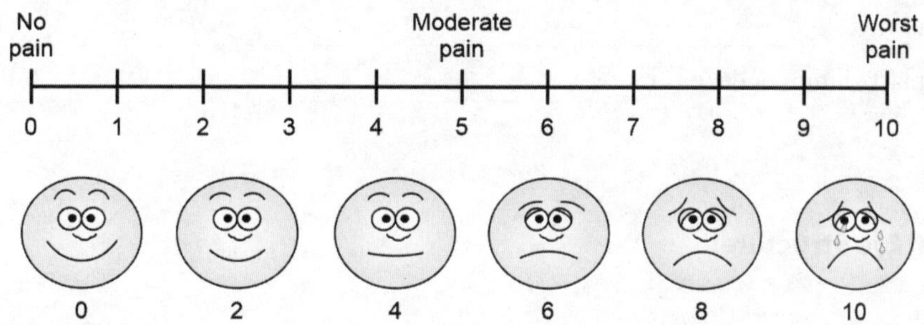

HEAD TO FEET EXAMINATION

HEAD

Inspection and Palpation:

- Hair (distribution/color/clean dry, etc.) ____________
- Any abrasions/wound/any device: ____________
- Scalp (clean, dandruff, pediculosis, etc.): ____________
- Size, shape and configuration: ____________
- Any involuntary movements: ____________

FACE

Inspection and Palpation:

- Shape, movement, expression and skin: ____________
- On palpation of temporal artery: ____________
- Palpation of temporomandibular joint (TMJ): ____________

NECK

Inspection:

- Position, symmetry, lump or mass: ____________
- Movement of neck structure: ____________
- Cervical vertebrae: ____________

Palpation:

- Trachea (position/mass): ____________
- Thyroid gland (landmark, lump, node, etc.): ____________

EYE (VISION)

Inspection of External Eye Structure:

- Eyelids and eyelashes: ____________
- Lid margin (ptosis retracted lid margin): ____________

- Ability to close eyelids: ____________________
- Any redness, swelling, discharge or lesion: ____________________
- Position alignment of the eyeball in the socket: ____________________
- Bulbar conjunctiva and sclera: ____________________
- Cornea and lens: ____________________
- Iris and pupil: ____________________
- Pupillary reaction to light: ____________________

Internal Eye Structure (Use Ophthalmoscope):

- Red reflects (round, regular border/black spots, etc.) ____________________
- Optic disc: ____________________
- Any foreign body, wound laceration, edema: ____________________

EAR (HEARING)

External Ear Structure

Inspection:

- Use of ear hearing aids: ____________________
- Appearance of auricle, tragus, lobule (size/position/color/discharge, etc.): ____________________

Palpation:

- Auricle and mastoids process (pain/tenderness): ____________________

Internal Ear Structure

Inspection:

- Auditory canal (color/earwax/any nodule): ____________________
- Tympanic membrane eardrum (color, shape, consistency, etc.): ____________________

Hearing and Equilibrium Test

- Whisper test: ____________________
- Weber's test: ____________________
- Rinne test: ____________________
- Romberg test: ____________________

MOUTH, THROAT AND NOSE

Mouth

Inspection and palpation:

- Lips (consistency/color): ______
- Teeth (no. of teeth present/color/condition, etc.): ______
- Gums (color/consistency/lesion/mass, etc.): ______
- Ventral surface of tongue (color/lesion, etc.): ______
- Wharton ducts (color, swelling or pain, etc.): ______
- Sides of tongue: ______
- Strength of tongue: ______
- Hard and soft palate and uvula (color/consistency/lesion, etc.): ______
- Odor from mouth (any foul odor): ______
- Uvula (position/color): ______
- Tonsils (color/size/any lesion or exudate, etc.): ______
- Posterior pharyngeal wall (color/any lesion or exudate, etc.): ______

Throat

Inspection:

- Inspect for nasal flaring and pursed lip breathing: ______
- Observe color of face, lips and chest: ______
- Inspect color of face, lips and chest: ______
- Inspect color and shape of nails: ______
- Patient is on: room air/oxygen/BiPAP/ventilator: ______
- If no O_2 support: Flow rate: ______ Mode: ______
- Endotracheal tube (present/absent) size: ______
- Respiratory pattern: ______

Nose

Inspection:

- External nose: ______
- Olfactory sense: ______
- Nasal septum: ______

POSTERIOR THORAX

Inspection:

- Scapula and spinous process (symmetry, shape, etc.): ____________
- Use of accessory muscle (trapezius/shoulder): ____________
- Sitting position: ____________

Palpation:

- Sensation and tenderness (warm/cold/sensation/pain/lesion/mass, etc.): ____________
- Crepitus: ____________
- Tactile fremitus (equal bilaterally): ____________
- Assess chest expansion: ____________

Percussion:

- Tone (resonance/hyperresonance): ____________
- Diaphragmatic excursion (normally 3–5 cm): ____________

Auscultation:

- Breathing sound heard (normal/abnormal, e.g., crackles/rhonchi/wheezes/pleural friction/rub/stridor/any other, etc.): ____________

Breathing sound at:

- Vesicular: ____________
- Bronchial: ____________
- Bronchovesicular: ____________
- Adventitious sound (present/absent): ____________

ANTERIOR THORAX

Inspection:

- Shape and configuration (symmetry/shape, etc.): ____________
- Ratio of anteroposterior verses transverse diameter (normal 1:2): ____________
- Position of sternum: ____________
- Sternal retraction: ____________
- Slope of the ribs: ____________
- Quality of accessory muscles (spermatoid/rectus abdominis, etc.): ____________

- Intercostal space (retraction/bulging): ______
- Use of accessory muscles (sternomastoid rectus abdominis): ______

Palpation:

- Sensation and tenderness (warm/cold/sensation/lesion/mass, etc.): ______
- Crepitus: ______
- Tactile fremitus (equal bilaterally): ______
- Assess chest expansion: ______

Percussion:

- Tone (resonance/hyperresonance): ______
- Diaphragmatic excursion (normally 3–5 cm): ______

Auscultation:

Breathing sound heard (normal/abnormal—e.g., crackles/rhonchi/wheezes/pleural friction/rub/stridor/any other, etc.):

______

Breathing sound at:

- Vesicular: ______
- Bronchial: ______
- Bronchovesicular: ______
- Adventitious sound (present/absent): ______
- Anterior thorax: ______
- Inspection: ______
- Shape and configuration (system/shape, etc.): ______
- Ratio of anteroposterior verses transverse diameter (normal 1:2): ______
- Position of sternum: ______
- Sternal retraction: ______
- Slope of the ribs: ______
- Quality and pattern of respiration: ______
- Intercostal space: (retraction/bulging): ______
- Use of accessory muscle (sternomastoid/rectus abdominis): ______

Palpation:

- Sensation and tenderness (warm/cold sensation/pain/lesion/mass, etc.): ______

- Crepitus: ______
- Tactile fremitus (equal bilaterally): ______
- Assess the chest expansion: ______

Percussion:

- Tone (resonance/hyperresonance): ______
- Diaphragmatic excursion (normally 3–5 cm): ______

Auscultation:

- Breathing sound heard (normal/abnormal, crackles/wheezes/pleural friction/rub/stridor/any other, etc.):
______
- Breathing sound at: ______
- Vesicular: ______
- Bronchial: ______
- Bronchovesicular: ______
- Adventitious sound (present/absent): ______

CHEST INSPECTION

- Size and symmetry: ______
- Color and texture: ______
- Superficial venous pattern: ______
- Areola (color/size/shape/texture): ______
- Nipple (size/direction/discharge/lesion, etc.) ______
- Retraction or dimpling:

FEMALE BREAST

Palpation:

- Tenderness and temperature: ______
- Mass (size/location/shape, etc.): ______
- Nipple (discharge): ______
- Scar (mastectomy/lumpectomy): ______

AXILLA

Inspection and Palpation:

- Mass/tenderness/lesion, etc.: ____________________

MALE BREAST

Areolas, Nipple, and Axilla

Inspection and palpation:

- Any swelling include/nodule/discharge, etc.: ____________________

NECK

Inspection:

- Jugular venous pulses: ____________________

Auscultation and Palpation:

- Auscultate carotid artery (bruit/blowing/swishing sound): ____________________
- Palpate carotid artery (elasticity/thrillers): ____________________

HEART (PERICARDIUM)

Inspection:

- Pulsation (visible location): ____________________

Palpation:

- Apical impulses (present/absent/location): ____________________

Auscultation:

- Rate (per minute): Regular/irregular rhythm: ____________________
- S1 (lub) and S2 (dub) sound: ____________________
- Extra heart sound: ____________________

ARMS

Inspection:

- Color, size, venous pattern and edema: ____________________

Palpation:

- Fingers, hands, arms and warmth: ______
- Capillary refill time: ______
- Radial pulse (elasticity and strength): ______
- Ulnar pulse (present/absent): ______
- Brachial pulse (strength): ______
- Allen test: ______

LEGS

Inspection, Palpation and Auscultation:

- Distribution of hair: ______
- Any lesions or ulcer: ______
- Edema with characteristics: ______
- Varicosities temperature of feet and legs: ______
- On palpation of superficial inguinal lymph nodes: ______
- On palpation superficial pulse (amplifier and strength): ______
- On auscultation of femoral pulse (amplitude and strength): ______
- On palpation of popliteal pulse: ______
- On palpation of dorsalis pedis pulse (strong/weak/absent): ______
- On palpation posterior tibia pulses (strong/weak/absent: ______

ABDOMEN

Inspection:

- Color of skin: ______
- Vascularity of the skin: ______
- Presence of scar: ______
- Assess for lesions and rashes: ______
- Observe for umbilical for skin color, location and contour: ______
- Abdominal contour (flat/rounded/scaphoid): ______
- Symmetry: ______
- Aortic pulsation: ______
- Peristaltic waves: ______
- Observable wave: ______

Auscultation:

Note: While doing the assessment of abdomen, auscultation is done before percussion and palpation, as their steps may alter the bowel sound.

- Bowel sound (intensity, pitch and frequency): ____________________
- Vascular sound (presence or absence of bruit sound): ____________________
- Venous rub over the spleen and liver: ____________________
- Friction rub over the spleen and liver: ____________________

Percussion:

- Percuss for tone (tympani and dull sound at different locations): ____________________
- The span or height of the liver: ____________________
- Spleen: ____________________
- Blunt percussion to find tenderness and muscular resistance: ____________________
- Deep palpation at all 4 quadrants to delineate abdominal organs and detect subtle masses: ____________________
- Assess for masses (in all quadrants): ____________________
- Umbilicus and surroundings: ____________________
- Liver (usually not palpable): ____________________
- Spleen (rarely palpable at left costal margin): ____________________
- Kidney (usually not palpable): ____________________
- Urinary bladder: ____________________

Special Test:

- Ascites (shifting dullness, fluid wave, etc.) ____________________
- Appendicitis (rebound tenderness, psoas sign, obturator sign, hypersensitivity test): ____________________

GAIT

Inspection:

- Patient's ability to walk and move around: ____________________
- Foot position, posture and arm swing during walk: ____________________
- Temporomandibular joint—inspection and palpation: ____________________
- Sternoclavicular joint—inspection and palpation: ____________________
- Cervical, thoracic and lumbar vertebra—inspection and palpation: ____________________

Movement of Cervical Spine:

- Flexion and hyperextension: ____________________
- Lateral bending: ____________________
- Rotation: ____________________

Movement of Thoracic and Lumbar Spine:

- Flexion and extension: ____________________
- Lateral bending: ____________________
- Rotation: ____________________
- Measure leg length: ____________________
- Straight leg test: ____________________

SHOULDER AND ARM

Inspection and Palpation:

- Assess for symmetry, color, swelling and masses: ____________________

Movement:

- Flexion and hyperextension: ____________________
- Adduction and abduction: ____________________
- External and internal rotation: ____________________

ELBOW

Inspection and Palpation:

- Assess size, shape, deformities, redness or swelling: ____________________

Movement:

- Flexion and extension: ____________________
- Supination and pronation: ____________________
- External and pronation: ____________________

WRIST

Inspection and Palpation:

- Assess size, shape symmetry, color, swelling: ____________________

- Presence of tenderness and nodules: ______
- Any tenderness in anatomical snuffbox: ______

Movement:

- Flexion and extension: ______
- Radial and ulnar deviation: ______

- Carpal tunnel syndrome: ______
- Phalen's test: ______
- Tinel's test: ______
- Flick test: ______
- Test for thumb weakness: ______

HANDS AND FINGERS

Inspection and Palpation:

- Assess size, shape symmetry, color, swelling: ______
- Palpate for tenderness, swelling bony prominence, nodules or crepitus: ______

Movement:

- Abduction and adduction: ______
- Flexion hyperextension: ______
- Internal and external hip rotation: ______

KNEE

Inspection and Palpation:

- Assess size, shape symmetry, swelling, deformities and alignment: ______
- On palpation knee (tenderness, warmth, consciousness, consistency nodule): ______

Movement:

- Flexion and hyperextension: ______
- Ballottement test: ______
- Mercury test: ______

ANKLES AND FEET

Inspection and Palpation:

- Assess patient in sitting, standing and walking for position, alignment, shape and skin of toe and feet: ______________
- Palpation of ankles and feet (tenderness, heat, swelling or nodule, pain): ______________
- Metatarsophalangeal joint (pain/tenderness): ______________

Movement:

- Dorsiflexion and plantarflexion of foot and ankle: ______________
- Eversion and inversion: ______________
- Abduction and adduction: ______________
- Flexion and extension: ______________

Reflexes:

	Biceps	Triceps	Brachioradialis	Patellar (quadriceps)	Achilles	Ankle clonus
Right side						
Left side						

Superficial Reflexes:

- Abdominal reflex: ______________
- Cremasteric reflex in male patient: ______________
- Test for meningeal irritation: ______________
- Brudziński's sign: ______________
- Kernig's sign: ______________

MALE GENITALIA

Penis

Inspection:

- Urinary catheter (present/absent): ____________________
- Inspect the base part of penis, pubic hairs, skin of the shaft, foreskin, glans: ____________________

Palpation:

- Palpate the shape for tenderness, pain, discharge, etc.____________________

Scrotum

Inspection:

- Inspect the shape, tenderness, and skin scrotum: ____________________

INGUINAL AREA

Inspection:

- Inspect the inguinal femoral areas for any bulge: ____________________

Palpation:

- Palpate on both side of inguinal area for lymph node, masses or bulging, femoral hernia: ____________________

____

FEMALE GENITALIA

External Genitalia

Inspection:

- Urinary catheter (present/absent): ____________________
- Assess the mons pubis, inguinal lymph, labia majora and perineum: ____________________
- Inspect the labia minora, clitoris, urethral meatus and vaginal opening: ____________________

Palpation:

- Bartholin gland (swelling, pain, discharge): ____________________
- Urethra (discharge, tenderness): ____________________

Internal Genitalia

Inspection:

- Observe the size and angle of vaginal opening: ____________________
- Assess vaginal musculature: ____________________
- Inspection of cervix (smoothness, color): ____________________
- Assess the vagina (redness, lesion, color, discharge): ____________________
- Bimanual examination (tenderness, lesion, pain): ____________________

Anus and Rectum

Inspection:

- Insect and opening area for lump, ulcer, lesion, rashes, redness, fissures, thickness of skin: ____________________
- Assess Valsalva maneuver: ____________________
- Assess sacrococcygeal area for swelling, redness, dimpling or hair, etc.: ____________________

Palpation:

- **Anus:** Any sphincter tightness, bleeding, pain, etc. ____________________
- **Rectum:** Presence of smoothness, tenderness, nodules, irregularities, etc.: ____________________
- **Prostate gland:** (normally nontender and rubbery): ____________________
- Inspect stool, if available: ____________________

INVESTIGATIONS

BLOOD/PATHOLOGICAL INVESTIGATIONS

Investigations	Normal values	Patient investigations values			Remark
		Date	Date	Date	
HEMATOLOGY					
Hemoglobin	12.5–17.5 g/dL				
RBC	4.50–6.0 × 10^6/mL				
PCV	35.0–50.4%				
MCV	80.0–99.9 fl				
MCH	27.0–31.0 pg.				
MCHC	33.0–37.0 g/dL				
Total WBC	4000–11000/cumm				
DLC: Polymorphs	40–75%				
Lymphocytes	20–40%				
Eosinophil	01–06%				
Monocytes	02–08%				
Basophil	00–01%				
Malaria parasite					
Smear: Normal					
Platelet count	1.5–4.5 lakhs/cumm				
ESR	Up to 15 mm at 1 hour				
AEC	40–440/cumm				
Retic count	0.5–2.5%				
Prothrombin time					
INR					
PTTK					
Bleeding time	1–5 minutes				
Clotting time	3–8 minutes				
Urine: Appearance					
Reaction					

Investigations	Normal values	Patient investigations values			Remark
		Date	Date	Date	
Albumin					
Sugar					
Acetone					
Bile salt/pigments					
Pus cells					
RBCs					
Others					
SEROLOGY: HIV					
HBsAg					
BIOCHEMISTRY					
Blood sugar fasting	70–110 mg/dL				
Postprandial	90–160 mg/dL				
Random	90–160 mg/dL				
HbA1c	4.2–6.2 mg/dL				
Blood urea	14–50 mg/dL				
Serum creatinine	0.6–1.4 mg/dL				
Uric acid	M: 2.7–7.7 mg/dL F: 2.4–5.7 mg/dL				
CPK	Up to 190 IU/L				
CPK MB	Up to 40 IU /L				
SGOT	Up to 40 IU/L				
LDH	Up to 450 IU /L				
Serum sodium	134–148 mEq /L				
Serum potassium	3.5–5.6 mEq/L				
Serum calcium	8.1–10.4 mg/dL				
Serum phosphorous	2.5–4.5 mg/dL				
Serum magnesium	1.8–2.6 mg/dL				
LIPID: Total cholesterol	Up to 200 mg/dL				
HDL cholesterol	40–60 mg/dL				
Serum triglycerides	Up to 150 mg/dL				
LDL cholesterol	Up to 100 mg/dL				

Investigations	Normal values	Patient investigations values			Remark
		Date	Date	Date	
LFT: Total protein	6.0–7.8 g/dL				
Albumin	3.2–4.5 g/dL				
Globulin	2.3–3.5 g/dL				
Bilirubin total	Up to 1.2 mg/dL				
Bilirubin direct	Up to 0.25 mg/dL				
SGPT	Up to 40 IU/L				
Alkaline phosphates	Up to 150 IU/L				
Serum digoxin	0.8–2.0 ng/mL				
Serum amylase	25–125 U/L				
SEROLOGY					
RA:					
CRP:					
ASO:					
TROP- T					

OTHER DIAGNOSTIC INVESTIGATIONS:

Ultrasonography (USG): (abdomen/pelvis/kidney/urethra/bladder (kub) etc.):

____

X-ray: (abdomen/pelvis/kidney/urethra/bladder (KUB) etc.):

____

Computer tomography (CT scan):

____

Magnetic resonance imagination: (MRI):

____

Any other:

____

MEDICATION

Sl. no.	Name of medication, route, dose	Action	Indication	Contraindication	Side effects	Nurses responsibility

PATIENT QUESTION: FEEDBACK

Question	Patient feedback
Student nurse: **Patient:**	

SUMMARY

BIBLIOGRAPHY/REFERENCES

(Write bibliography in the Vancouver style)

EVALUATION CRITERIA FOR HISTORY TAKING

Name of the Student: ______________________ **Date:**

Clinical Area: ______________________ **Diagnosis:** ______________________

Sl. no.	Criteria	Allotted marks	Obtained marks
1.	History collection	3	
2.	Physical examination	3	
3.	Drug study	2	
4.	Nursing assessment	2	
5.	Prioritize the nursing diagnosis	5	
6.	Nursing care plan on 5 need-based nursing diagnosis	5	
7.	Prognosis of patient	1	
8.	Nurses notes	2	
9.	Bibliography/References	2	
Total		**25**	

Remarks: ______________________

____

Signature of the Student

Signature of the Evaluator

HISTORY TAKING–2 (SURGICAL)

BIOGRAPHICAL DATA OF PATIENT

Name of the Patient: ______________________ Age: ________ Gender: ____________

Date of Health History Collection: ______________________ Date of Admission: ____________

Hospital/IP No: ______________________ Language Spoken: ____________

Marital Status: ____________ Educational Status: ____________ Religion: ____________

Occupation: ______________________ Provisional Diagnosis: ____________

Treatment under Doctor: ______________________

Name of the procedure (if surgery/procedure done): ______________________

CHIEF COMPLAINTS

____

____

____

____

____

HISTORY OF PRESENT ILLNESS

____

____

____

____

____

PAST MEDICAL HISTORY

- Past illness and treatment (birth problem/childhood illness/immunization history): History of blood transfusion:
- Any allergic history (food/medication/other):
- Any other relevant (physical/psychological or mental illness):
- Previous hospitalization:

SOCIOECONOMIC STATUS

FAMILY HISTORY OF ANY ILLNESS

Family Tree Diagram:

Genogram Key	
Female	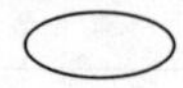
Male	
Patient	
Deceased	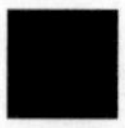 OR 
Cause of death	( )
Adoption (vertical)	| ====
Consanguinity	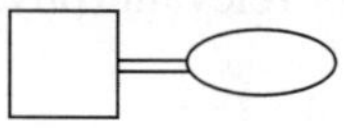

(For reference)

History of chronic illness such as: (diabetes mellitus, hypertension, coronary artery disease, renal disease, psychiatric illness, cancer, etc.): ______________________________

____

____

History of any recent death in the family: ______________________________

____

____

History of any hereditary disease or communicable disease in the family: ______________________________

____

PERSONAL HISTORY

- Personal hygiene: ______________________________

  ____

- Dietary history (veg/non-veg/meal pattern, any practice): ______________________________

  ____

- Elimination pattern: ____________________

____

- Physical activities and exercises: ____________________

____

- Work pattern (type, level of job satisfaction, work stress, etc.): ____________________

____

- Sleeping/rest pattern: ____________________

____

- Hobbies: ____________________

____

- Use of any addictive substances: ____________________

____

- Relationship with patient, friends, significant others: ____________________

____

- Social activities and religious activities: ____________________

____

PHYSICAL EXAMINATION

GENERAL APPEARANCE

- **Level of consciousness**: (consciousness/unconsciousness/semi-consciousness/coma/confused, etc.): ______________________________
- Orientation (time/place/person): ______________________________
- Mood: ______________________________
- Activity: ______________________________
- Body built: ______________________________

Weight: ______________ **Height** (inches/cm): ______________ **BMI** (weight (kg)/height in meter^2): ______________

VITAL SIGNS

Day/Date	Temperature (In °F/°C)	Pulse (beats/min)	Respiration (breaths/min)	Blood pressure (mm Hg)	Pain score on VAS

VISUAL ANALOGUE PAIN (VAS) SCALE

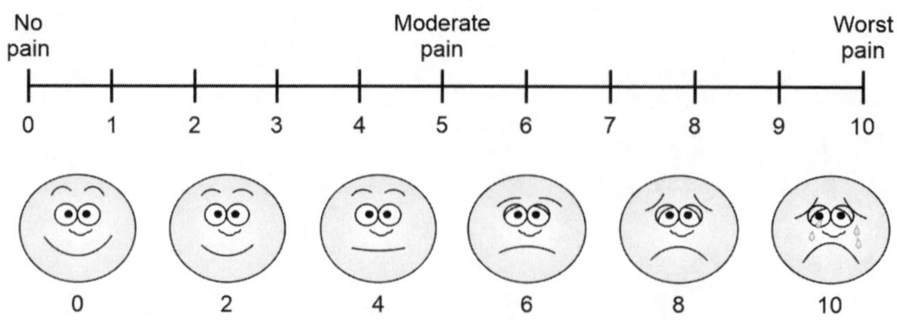

HEAD TO FEET EXAMINATION

HEAD

Inspection and Palpation:

- Hair (distribution/color/clean dry, etc.) ______
- Any abrasions/wound/any device: ______
- Scalp (clean, dandruff, pediculosis, etc.): ______
- Size, shape and configuration: ______
- Any involuntary movements: ______

FACE

Inspection and Palpation:

- Shape, movement, expression and skin: ______
- On palpation of temporal artery: ______
- Palpation of temporomandibular joint (TMJ): ______

NECK

Inspection:

- Position, symmetry, lump or mass: ______
- Movement of neck structure: ______
- Cervical vertebrae: ______

Palpation:

- Trachea (position/mass): ______
- Thyroid gland (landmark, lump, node, etc.): ______

EYE (VISION)

Inspection of External Eye Structure:

- Eyelids and eyelashes: ______
- Lid margin (ptosis retracted lid margin): ______

- Ability to close eyelids: ____________
- Any redness, swelling, discharge or lesion: ____________
- Position alignment of the eyeball in the socket: ____________
- Bulbar conjunctiva and sclera: ____________
- Cornea and lens: ____________
- Iris and pupil: ____________
- Pupillary reaction to light: ____________

Internal Eye Structure (Use Ophthalmoscope):

- Red reflects (round, regular border/black spots, etc.) ____________
- Optic disc: ____________
- Any foreign body, wound laceration, edema: ____________

EAR (HEARING)

External Ear Structure

Inspection:

- Use of ear hearing aids: ____________
- Appearance of auricle, tragus, lobule (size/position/color/discharge, etc.): ____________

Palpation:

- Auricle and mastoids process (pain/tenderness): ____________

Internal Ear Structure

Inspection:

- Auditory canal (color/earwax/any nodule): ____________
- Tympanic membrane eardrum (color, shape, consistency, etc.): ____________

Hearing and Equilibrium Test:

- Whisper test: ____________
- Weber's test: ____________
- Rinne test: ____________
- Romberg test: ____________

MOUTH, THROAT AND NOSE

Mouth

Inspection and palpation:

- Lips (consistency/color): ____________________
- Teeth (no. of teeth present/color/condition, etc.): ____________________
- Gums (color/consistency/lesion/mass, etc.): ____________________
- Ventral surface of tongue (color/lesion, etc.): ____________________
- Wharton ducts (color, swelling or pain, etc.): ____________________
- Sides of tongue: ____________________
- Strength of tongue: ____________________
- Hard and soft palate and uvula (color/consistency/lesion, etc.): ____________________
- Odor from mouth (any foul odor): ____________________
- Uvula (position/color): ____________________
- Tonsils (color/size/any lesion or exudate, etc.): ____________________
- Posterior pharyngeal wall (color/any lesion or exudate, etc.): ____________________

Throat

Inspection:

- Inspect for nasal flaring and pursed lip breathing: ____________________
- Observe color of face, lips and chest: ____________________
- Inspect color of face, lips and chest: ____________________
- Inspect color and shape of nails: ____________________
- Patient is on: room air/oxygen/BiPAP/ventilator: ____________________
- If no O_2 support: Flow rate: ____________________ Mode: ____________________
- Endotracheal tube (present/absent) size: ____________________
- Respiratory pattern: ____________________

Nose

Inspection:

- External nose: ____________________
- Olfactory sense: ____________________
- Nasal septum: ____________________

POSTERIOR THORAX

Inspection:

- Scapula and spinous process (symmetry, shape, etc.): __________
- Use of accessory muscle (trapezius/shoulder): __________
- Sitting position: __________

Palpation:

- Sensation and tenderness (warm/cold/sensation/pain/lesion/mass, etc.): __________
- Crepitus: __________
- Tactile fremitus (equal bilaterally): __________
- Assess chest expansion: __________

Percussion:

- Tone (resonance/hyperresonance): __________
- Diaphragmatic excursion (normally 3–5 cm): __________

Auscultation:

- Breathing sound heard (normal/abnormal, e.g., crackles/rhonchi/wheezes/pleural friction/rub/stridor/any other, etc.): __________

Breathing sound at:

- Vesicular: __________
- Bronchial: __________
- Bronchovesicular: __________
- Adventitious sound (present/absent): __________

ANTERIOR THORAX

Inspection:

- Shape and configuration (symmetry/shape, etc.): __________
- Ratio of anteroposterior verses transverse diameter (normal 1:2): __________
- Position of sternum: __________
- Sternal retraction: __________
- Slope of the ribs: __________
- Quality of accessory muscles (spermatoid/rectus abdominis, etc.): __________

- Intercostal space (retraction/bulging): ____________________
- Use of accessory muscles (sternomastoid rectus abdominis): ____________________

Palpation:

- Sensation and tenderness (warm/cold/sensation/lesion/mass, etc.): ____________________
- Crepitus: ____________________
- Tactile fremitus (equal bilaterally): ____________________
- Assess chest expansion: ____________________

Percussion:

- Tone (resonance/hyperresonance): ____________________
- Diaphragmatic excursion (normally 3–5 cm): ____________________

Auscultation:

Breathing sound heard (normal/abnormal—e.g., crackles/rhonchi/wheezes/pleural friction/rub/stridor/any other, etc.): ____________________

Breathing sound at:

- Vesicular: ____________________
- Bronchial: ____________________
- Bronchovesicular: ____________________
- Adventitious sound (present/absent): ____________________
- Anterior thorax: ____________________
- Inspection: ____________________
- Shape and configuration (system/shape, etc.): ____________________
- Ratio of anteroposterior verses transverse diameter (normal 1:2): ____________________
- Position of sternum: ____________________
- Sternal retraction: ____________________
- Slope of the ribs: ____________________
- Quality and pattern of respiration: ____________________
- Intercostal space: (retraction/bulging): ____________________
- Use of accessory muscle (sternomastoid/rectus abdominis): ____________________

Palpation:

- Sensation and tenderness (warm/cold sensation/pain/lesion/mass, etc.): ____________________

- Crepitus: ______
- Tactile fremitus (equal bilaterally): ______
- Assess the chest expansion: ______

Percussion:

- Tone (resonance/hyperresonance): ______
- Diaphragmatic excursion (normally 3–5 cm): ______

Auscultation:

- Breathing sound heard (normal/abnormal, crackles/wheezes/pleural friction/rub/stridor/any other, etc.):
  ______
- Breathing sound at: ______
- Vesicular: ______
- Bronchial: ______
- Bronchovesicular: ______
- Adventitious sound (present/absent): ______

CHEST INSPECTION

- Size and symmetry: ______
- Color and texture: ______
- Superficial venous pattern: ______
- Areola (color/size/shape/texture): ______
- Nipple (size/direction/discharge/lesion, etc.) ______
- Retraction or dimpling:

FEMALE BREAST

Palpation:

- Tenderness and temperature: ______
- Mass (size/location/shape, etc.): ______
- Nipple (discharge): ______
- Scar (mastectomy/lumpectomy): ______

AXILLA

Inspection and Palpation:

- Mass/tenderness/lesion, etc.: ____________

MALE BREAST

Areolas, Nipple, and Axilla

Inspection and palpation:

- Any swelling include/nodule/discharge, etc.: ____________

NECK

Inspection:

- Jugular venous pulses: ____________

Auscultation and Palpation:

- Auscultate carotid artery (bruit/blowing/swishing sound): ____________
- Palpate carotid artery (elasticity/thrillers): ____________

HEART (PERICARDIUM)

Inspection:

- Pulsation (visible location): ____________

Palpation:

- Apical impulses (present/absent/location): ____________

Auscultation:

- Rate (per minute): Regular/irregular rhythm: ____________
- S1 (lub) and S2 (dub) sound: ____________
- Extra heart sound: ____________

ARMS

Inspection:

- Color, size, venous pattern and edema: ____________

Palpation:

- Fingers, hands, arms and warmth: ____________
- Capillary refill time: ____________
- Radial pulse (elasticity and strength): ____________
- Ulnar pulse (present/absent): ____________
- Brachial pulse (strength): ____________
- Allen test: ____________

LEGS

Inspection, Palpation and Auscultation:

- Distribution of hair: ____________
- Any lesions or ulcer: ____________
- Edema with characteristics: ____________
- Varicosities temperature of feet and legs: ____________
- On palpation of superficial inguinal lymph nodes: ____________
- On palpation superficial pulse (amplifier and strength): ____________
- On auscultation of femoral pulse (amplitude and strength): ____________
- On palpation of popliteal pulse: ____________
- On palpation of dorsalis pedis pulse (strong/weak/absent): ____________
- On palpation posterior tibia pulses (strong/weak/absent: ____________

ABDOMEN

Inspection:

- Color of skin: ____________
- Vascularity of the skin: ____________
- Presence of scar: ____________
- Assess for lesions and rashes: ____________
- Observe for umbilical for skin color, location and contour: ____________
- Abdominal contour (flat/rounded/scaphoid): ____________
- Symmetry: ____________
- Aortic pulsation: ____________
- Peristaltic waves: ____________
- Observable wave: ____________

Auscultation:

Note: While doing the assessment of abdomen, auscultation is done before percussion and palpation, as their steps may alter the bowel sound.

- Bowel sound (intensity, pitch and frequency): ____________
- Vascular sound (presence or absence of bruit sound): ____________
- Venous rub over the spleen and liver: ____________
- Friction rub over the spleen and liver: ____________

Percussion:

- Percuss for tone (tympani and dull sound at different locations): ____________
- The span or height of the liver: ____________
- Spleen: ____________
- Blunt percussion to find tenderness and muscular resistance: ____________
- Deep palpation at all 4 quadrants to delineate abdominal organs and detect subtle masses: ____________
- Assess for masses (in all quadrants): ____________
- Umbilicus and surroundings: ____________
- Liver (usually not palpable): ____________
- Spleen (rarely palpable at left costal margin): ____________
- Kidney (usually not palpable): ____________
- Urinary bladder: ____________

Special Test:

- Ascites (shifting dullness, fluid wave, etc.) ____________
- Appendicitis (rebound tenderness, psoas sign, obturator sign, hypersensitivity test): ____________

GAIT

Inspection:

- Patient's ability to walk and move around: ____________
- Foot position, posture and arm swing during walk: ____________
- Temporomandibular joint—inspection and palpation: ____________
- Sternoclavicular joint—inspection and palpation: ____________
- Cervical, thoracic and lumbar vertebra—inspection and palpation: ____________

Movement of Cervical Spine:

- Flexion and hyperextension: ____
- Lateral bending: ____
- Rotation: ____

Movement of Thoracic and Lumbar Spine:

- Flexion and extension: ____
- Lateral bending: ____
- Rotation: ____
- Measure leg length: ____
- Straight leg test: ____

SHOULDER AND ARM

Inspection and Palpation:

- Assess for symmetry, color, swelling and masses: ____

Movement:

- Flexion and hyperextension: ____
- Adduction and abduction: ____
- External and internal rotation: ____

ELBOW

Inspection and Palpation:

- Assess size, shape, deformities, redness or swelling: ____

Movement:

- Flexion and extension: ____
- Supination and pronation: ____
- External and pronation: ____

WRIST

Inspection and Palpation:

- Assess size, shape symmetry, color, swelling: ____

- Presence of tenderness and nodules: ______
- Any tenderness in anatomical snuffbox: ______

Movement:

  - Flexion and extension: ______
  - Radial and ulnar deviation: ______

- Carpal tunnel syndrome: ______
- Phalen's test: ______
- Tinel's test: ______
- Flick test: ______
- Test for thumb weakness: ______

HANDS AND FINGERS

Inspection and Palpation:

- Assess size, shape symmetry, color, swelling: ______
- Palpate for tenderness, swelling bony prominence, nodules or crepitus: ______

Movement:

- Abduction and adduction: ______
- Flexion hyperextension: ______
- Internal and external hip rotation: ______

KNEE

Inspection and Palpation:

- Assess size, shape symmetry, swelling, deformities and alignment: ______
- On palpation knee (tenderness, warmth, consciousness, consistency nodule): ______

Movement:

- Flexion and hyperextension: ______
- Ballottement test: ______
- Mercury test: ______

ANKLES AND FEET

Inspection and Palpation:

- Assess patient in sitting, standing and walking for position, alignment, shape and skin of toe and feet: ____________
- Palpation of ankles and feet (tenderness, heat, swelling or nodule, pain): ____________
- Metatarsophalangeal joint (pain/tenderness): ____________

Movement:

- Dorsiflexion and plantarflexion of foot and ankle: ____________
- Eversion and inversion: ____________
- Abduction and adduction: ____________
- Flexion and extension: ____________

Reflexes:

	Biceps	Triceps	Brachioradialis	Patellar (quadriceps)	Achilles	Ankle clonus
Right side						
Left side						

Superficial Reflexes:

- Abdominal reflex: ____________
- Cremasteric reflex in male patient: ____________
- Test for meningeal irritation: ____________
- Brudziński's sign: ____________
- Kernig's sign: ____________

MALE GENITALIA

Penis

Inspection:

- Urinary catheter (present/absent): ______
- Inspect the base part of penis, pubic hairs, skin of the shaft, foreskin, glans: ______

Palpation:

- Palpate the shape for tenderness, pain, discharge, etc. ______

Scrotum

Inspection:

- Inspect the shape, tenderness, and skin scrotum: ______

INGUINAL AREA

Inspection:

- Inspect the inguinal femoral areas for any bulge: ______

Palpation:

- Palpate on both side of inguinal area for lymph node, masses or bulging, femoral hernia: ______

______

FEMALE GENITALIA

External Genitalia

Inspection:

- Urinary catheter (present/absent): ______
- Assess the mons pubis, inguinal lymph, labia majora and perineum: ______
- Inspect the labia minora, clitoris, urethral meatus and vaginal opening: ______

Palpation:

- Bartholin gland (swelling, pain, discharge): ______
- Urethra (discharge, tenderness): ______

Internal Genitalia

Inspection:

- Observe the size and angle of vaginal opening: ______
- Assess vaginal musculature: ______
- Inspection of cervix (smoothness, color): ______
- Assess the vagina (redness, lesion, color, discharge): ______
- Bimanual examination (tenderness, lesion, pain): ______

Anus and Rectum

Inspection:

- Insect and opening area for lump, ulcer, lesion, rashes, redness, fissures, thickness of skin: ______
- Assess Valsalva maneuver: ______
- Assess sacrococcygeal area for swelling, redness, dimpling or hair, etc.: ______

Palpation:

- **Anus:** Any sphincter tightness, bleeding, pain, etc. ______
- **Rectum:** Presence of smoothness, tenderness, nodules, irregularities, etc.: ______
- **Prostate gland:** (normally nontender and rubbery): ______
- Inspect stool, if available: ______

INVESTIGATIONS

BLOOD/PATHOLOGICAL INVESTIGATIONS

Investigations	Normal values	Patient investigations values			Remark
		Date	Date	Date	
HEMATOLOGY					
Hemoglobin	12.5–17.5 g/dL				
RBC	4.50–6.0 × 10^6/mL				
PCV	35.0–50.4%				
MCV	80.0–99.9 fl				
MCH	27.0–31.0 pg.				
MCHC	33.0–37.0 g/dL				
Total WBC	4000–11000/cumm				
DLC: Polymorphs	40–75%				
Lymphocytes	20–40%				
Eosinophil	01–06%				
Monocytes	02–08%				
Basophil	00–01%				
Malaria parasite					
Smear: Normal					
Platelet count	1.5–4.5 lakhs/cumm				
ESR	Up to 15 mm at 1 hour				
AEC	40–440/cumm				
Retic count	0.5–2.5%				
Prothrombin time					
INR					
PTTK					
Bleeding time	1–5 minutes				
Clotting time	3–8 minutes				
Urine: Appearance					
Reaction					
Albumin					

Investigations	Normal values	Patient investigations values			Remark
		Date	Date	Date	
Sugar					
Acetone					
Bile salt/pigments					
Pus cells					
RBCs					
Others					
SEROLOGY: HIV					
HBsAg					
BIOCHEMISTRY					
Blood sugar fasting	70–110 mg/dL				
Postprandial	90–160 mg/dL				
Random	90–160 mg/dL				
HbA1c	4.2–6.2 mg/dL				
Blood urea	14–50 mg/dL				
Serum creatinine	0.6–1.4 mg/dL				
Uric acid	M: 2.7–7.7 mg/dL F: 2.4–5.7 mg/dL				
CPK	Up to 190 IU/L				
CPK MB	Up to 40 IU /L				
SGOT	Up to 40 IU/L				
LDH	Up to 450 IU /L				
Serum sodium	134–148 mEq /L				
Serum potassium	3.5–5.6 mEq/L				
Serum calcium	8.1–10.4 mg/dL				
Serum phosphorous	2.5–4.5 mg/dL				
Serum magnesium	1.8–2.6 mg/dL				
LIPID: Total cholesterol	Up to 200 mg/dL				
HDL cholesterol	40–60 mg/dL				
Serum triglycerides	Up to 150 mg/dL				
LDL cholesterol	Up to 100 mg/dL				

Investigations	Normal values	Patient investigations values			Remark
		Date	Date	Date	
LFT: Total protein	6.0–7.8 g/dL				
Albumin	3.2–4.5 g/dL				
Globulin	2.3–3.5 g/dL				
Bilirubin total	Up to 1.2 mg/dL				
Bilirubin direct	Up to 0.25 mg/dL				
SGPT	Up to 40 IU/L				
Alkaline phosphates	Up to 150 IU/L				
Serum digoxin	0.8–2.0 ng/mL				
Serum amylase	25–125 U/L				
SEROLOGY					
RA:					
CRP:					
ASO:					
TROP- T					

OTHER DIAGNOSTIC INVESTIGATIONS:

Ultrasonography (USG): (abdomen/pelvis/kidney/urethra/bladder (kub) etc.):

____

X-ray: (abdomen/pelvis/kidney/urethra/bladder (KUB) etc.):

____

Computer tomography (CT scan):

____

Magnetic resonance imagination: (MRI):

____

Any other:

____

MEDICATION

Sl. no.	Name of medication, route, dose	Action	Indication	Contraindication	Side effects	Nurses responsibility

PATIENT QUESTION: FEEDBACK

Question	Patient feedback
Student nurse: **Patient:**	

SUMMARY

BIBLIOGRAPHY/REFERENCES

(Write bibliography in the Vancouver style)

EVALUATION CRITERIA FOR HISTORY TAKING

Name of the Student: ____________________ **Date:** __________

Clinical Area: ____________________ **Diagnosis:** __________

Sl. no.	Criteria	Allotted marks	Obtained marks
1.	History collection	3	
2.	Physical examination	3	
3.	Drug study	2	
4.	Nursing assessment	2	
5.	Prioritize the nursing diagnosis	5	
6.	Nursing care plan on 5 need-based nursing diagnosis	5	
7.	Prognosis of patient	1	
8.	Nurses notes	2	
9.	Bibliography/References	2	
Total		**25**	

Remarks: ____________________

Signature of the Student

Signature of the Evaluator

PHYSICAL EXAMINATION–1

BIOGRAPHICAL DATA OF PATIENT

Name of the Patient: ______________________ Age: ________ Gender: ____________

Date of Health History Collection: ______________________ Date of Admission: ____________

Hospital/IP No: ______________________ Language Spoken: ______________________

Marital Status: ____________ Educational Status: ____________ Religion: ____________

Occupation: ______________________ Provisional Diagnosis: ______________________

Treatment under Doctor: ____

Name of the procedure (if surgery/procedure done): ______________________

CHIEF COMPLAINTS

____

____

____

____

____

HISTORY OF PRESENT ILLNESS

____

____

____

____

____

PAST MEDICAL HISTORY

- Past illness and treatment (birth problem/childhood illness/immunization history): History of blood transfusion:
- Any allergic history (food/medication/other):
- Any other relevant (physical/psychological or mental illness):
- Previous hospitalization:

SOCIOECONOMIC STATUS

FAMILY HISTORY OF ANY ILLNESS

Family Tree Diagram:

Genogram Key	
Female	⬭
Male	□
Patient	↗
Deceased	■ OR ⬬
Cause of death	( )
Adoption (vertical)	|====
Consanguinity	□═⬭

(For reference)

History of chronic illness such as: (diabetes mellitus, hypertension, coronary artery disease, renal disease, psychiatric illness, cancer, etc.): ______________________________

____

____

History of any recent death in the family: ______________________________

____

____

History of any hereditary disease or communicable disease in the family: ______________________________

____

PERSONAL HISTORY

- Personal hygiene: ______________________________

  ____

- Dietary history (veg/non-veg/meal pattern, any practice): ______________________________

  ____

- Elimination pattern: ____________________

____

- Physical activities and exercises: ____________________

____

- Work pattern (type, level of job satisfaction, work stress, etc.): ____________________

____

- Sleeping/rest pattern: ____________________

____

- Hobbies: ____________________

____

- Use of any addictive substances: ____________________

____

- Relationship with patient, friends, significant others: ____________________

____

- Social activities and religious activities: ____________________

____

PHYSICAL EXAMINATION

GENERAL APPEARANCE

- **Level of consciousness**: (consciousness/unconsciousness/semi-consciousness/coma/confused, etc.):

  ____

- Orientation (time/place/person): ______________________________
- Mood: ______________________________
- Activity: ______________________________
- Body built: ______________________________

Weight: ____________ **Height** (inches/cm): ____________ **BMI** (weight (kg)/height in meter^2): ____________

VITAL SIGNS

Day/Date	Temperature (In °F/°C)	Pulse (beats/min)	Respiration (breaths/min)	Blood pressure (mm Hg)	Pain score on VAS

VISUAL ANALOGUE PAIN (VAS) SCALE

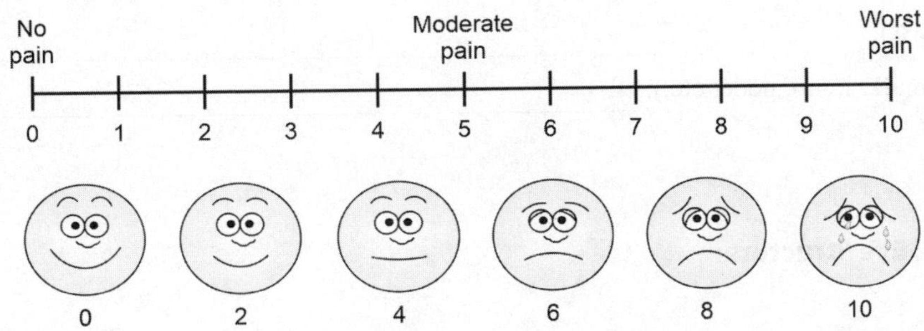

HEAD TO FEET EXAMINATION

HEAD

Inspection and Palpation:

- Hair (distribution/color/clean dry, etc.) ____________________
- Any abrasions/wound/any device: ____________________
- Scalp (clean, dandruff, pediculosis, etc.): ____________________
- Size, shape and configuration: ____________________
- Any involuntary movements: ____________________

FACE

Inspection and Palpation:

- Shape, movement, expression and skin: ____________________
- On palpation of temporal artery: ____________________
- Palpation of temporomandibular joint (TMJ): ____________________

NECK

Inspection:

- Position, symmetry, lump or mass: ____________________
- Movement of neck structure: ____________________
- Cervical vertebrae: ____________________

Palpation:

- Trachea (position/mass): ____________________
- Thyroid gland (landmark, lump, node, etc.): ____________________

EYE (VISION)

Inspection of External Eye Structure:

- Eyelids and eyelashes: ____________________
- Lid margin (ptosis retracted lid margin): ____________________

- Ability to close eyelids: ____________________
- Any redness, swelling, discharge or lesion: ____________________
- Position alignment of the eyeball in the socket: ____________________
- Bulbar conjunctiva and sclera: ____________________
- Cornea and lens: ____________________
- Iris and pupil: ____________________
- Pupillary reaction to light: ____________________

Internal Eye Structure (Use Ophthalmoscope):

- Red reflects (round, regular border/black spots, etc.): ____________________
- Optic disc: ____________________
- Any foreign body, wound laceration, edema: ____________________

EAR (HEARING)

External Ear Structure

Inspection:

- Use of ear hearing aids: ____________________
- Appearance of auricle, tragus, lobule (size/position/color/discharge, etc.): ____________________

Palpation:

- Auricle and mastoids process (pain/tenderness): ____________________

Internal Ear Structure

Inspection:

- Auditory canal (color/earwax/any nodule): ____________________
- Tympanic membrane eardrum (color, shape, consistency, etc.): ____________________

Hearing and Equilibrium Test:

- Whisper test: ____________________
- Weber's test: ____________________
- Rinne test: ____________________
- Romberg test: ____________________

MOUTH, THROAT AND NOSE

Mouth

Inspection and palpation:

- Lips (consistency/color): ____________
- Teeth (no. of teeth present/color/condition, etc.): ____________
- Gums (color/consistency/lesion/mass, etc.): ____________
- Ventral surface of tongue (color/lesion, etc.): ____________
- Wharton ducts (color, swelling or pain, etc.): ____________
- Sides of tongue: ____________
- Strength of tongue: ____________
- Hard and soft palate and uvula (color/consistency/lesion, etc.): ____________
- Odor from mouth (any foul odor): ____________
- Uvula (position/color): ____________
- Tonsils (color/size/any lesion or exudate, etc.): ____________
- Posterior pharyngeal wall (color/any lesion or exudate, etc.): ____________

Throat

Inspection:

- Inspect for nasal flaring and pursed lip breathing: ____________
- Observe color of face, lips and chest: ____________
- Inspect color of face, lips and chest: ____________
- Inspect color and shape of nails: ____________
- Patient is on: room air/oxygen/BiPAP/ventilator: ____________
- If no O_2 support: Flow rate: ____________ Mode: ____________
- Endotracheal tube (present/absent) size: ____________
- Respiratory pattern: ____________

Nose

Inspection:

- External nose: ____________
- Olfactory sense: ____________
- Nasal septum: ____________

POSTERIOR THORAX

Inspection:

- Scapula and spinous process (symmetry, shape, etc.): ______
- Use of accessory muscle (trapezius/shoulder): ______
- Sitting position: ______

Palpation:

- Sensation and tenderness (warm/cold/sensation/pain/lesion/mass, etc.): ______
- Crepitus: ______
- Tactile fremitus (equal bilaterally): ______
- Assess chest expansion: ______

Percussion:

- Tone (resonance/hyperresonance): ______
- Diaphragmatic excursion (normally 3–5 cm): ______

Auscultation:

- Breathing sound heard (normal/abnormal, e.g., crackles/rhonchi/wheezes/pleural friction/rub/stridor/any other, etc.):

______

Breathing sound at:

- Vesicular: ______
- Bronchial: ______
- Bronchovesicular: ______
- Adventitious sound (present/absent): ______

ANTERIOR THORAX

Inspection:

- Shape and configuration (symmetry/shape, etc.): ______
- Ratio of anteroposterior verses transverse diameter (normal 1:2): ______
- Position of sternum: ______
- Sternal retraction: ______
- Slope of the ribs: ______
- Quality of accessory muscles (spermatoid/rectus abdominis, etc.): ______

- Intercostal space (retraction/bulging): __________
- Use of accessory muscles (sternomastoid rectus abdominis): __________

Palpation:

- Sensation and tenderness (warm/cold/sensation/lesion/mass, etc.): __________
- Crepitus: __________
- Tactile fremitus (equal bilaterally): __________
- Assess chest expansion: __________

Percussion:

- Tone (resonance/hyperresonance): __________
- Diaphragmatic excursion (normally 3–5 cm): __________

Auscultation:

Breathing sound heard (normal/abnormal—e.g., crackles/rhonchi/wheezes/pleural friction/rub/stridor/any other, etc.):

____

Breathing sound at:

- Vesicular: __________
- Bronchial: __________
- Bronchovesicular: __________
- Adventitious sound (present/absent): __________
- Anterior thorax: __________
- Inspection: __________
- Shape and configuration (system/shape, etc.): __________
- Ratio of anteroposterior verses transverse diameter (normal 1:2): __________
- Position of sternum: __________
- Sternal retraction: __________
- Slope of the ribs: __________
- Quality and pattern of respiration: __________
- Intercostal space: (retraction/bulging): __________
- Use of accessory muscle (sternomastoid/rectus abdominis): __________

Palpation:

- Sensation and tenderness (warm/cold sensation/pain/lesion/mass, etc.): __________

- Crepitus: ______
- Tactile fremitus (equal bilaterally): ______
- Assess the chest expansion: ______

Percussion:

- Tone (resonance/hyperresonance): ______
- Diaphragmatic excursion (normally 3–5 cm): ______

Auscultation:

- Breathing sound heard (normal/abnormal, crackles/wheezes/pleural friction/rub/stridor/any other, etc.):
  ______
- Breathing sound at: ______
- Vesicular: ______
- Bronchial: ______
- Bronchovesicular: ______
- Adventitious sound (present/absent): ______

CHEST INSPECTION

- Size and symmetry: ______
- Color and texture: ______
- Superficial venous pattern: ______
- Areola (color/size/shape/texture): ______
- Nipple (size/direction/discharge/lesion, etc.) ______
- Retraction or dimpling:

FEMALE BREAST

Palpation:

- Tenderness and temperature: ______
- Mass (size/location/shape, etc.): ______
- Nipple (discharge): ______
- Scar (mastectomy/lumpectomy): ______

AXILLA

Inspection and Palpation:

- Mass/tenderness/lesion, etc.: ______________________

MALE BREAST

Areolas, Nipple, and Axilla

Inspection and palpation:

- Any swelling include/nodule/discharge, etc.: ______________________

NECK

Inspection:

- Jugular venous pulses: ______________________

Auscultation and Palpation:

- Auscultate carotid artery (bruit/blowing/swishing sound): ______________________
- Palpate carotid artery (elasticity/thrillers): ______________________

HEART (PERICARDIUM)

Inspection:

- Pulsation (visible location): ______________________

Palpation:

- Apical impulses (present/absent/location): ______________________

Auscultation:

- Rate (per minute): Regular/irregular rhythm: ______________________
- S1 (lub) and S2 (dub) sound: ______________________
- Extra heart sound: ______________________

ARMS

Inspection:

- Color, size, venous pattern and edema: ______________________

Palpation:

- Fingers, hands, arms and warmth: ____
- Capillary refill time: ____
- Radial pulse (elasticity and strength): ____
- Ulnar pulse (present/absent): ____
- Brachial pulse (strength): ____
- Allen test: ____

LEGS

Inspection, Palpation and Auscultation:

- Distribution of hair: ____
- Any lesions or ulcer: ____
- Edema with characteristics: ____
- Varicosities temperature of feet and legs: ____
- On palpation of superficial inguinal lymph nodes: ____
- On palpation superficial pulse (amplifier and strength): ____
- On auscultation of femoral pulse (amplitude and strength): ____
- On palpation of popliteal pulse: ____
- On palpation of dorsalis pedis pulse (strong/weak/absent): ____
- On palpation posterior tibia pulses (strong/weak/absent: ____

ABDOMEN

Inspection:

- Color of skin: ____
- Vascularity of the skin: ____
- Presence of scar: ____
- Assess for lesions and rashes: ____
- Observe for umbilical for skin color, location and contour: ____
- Abdominal contour (flat/rounded/scaphoid): ____
- Symmetry: ____
- Aortic pulsation: ____
- Peristaltic waves: ____
- Observable wave: ____

Auscultation:

Note: While doing the assessment of abdomen, auscultation is done before percussion and palpation, as their steps may alter the bowel sound.

- Bowel sound (intensity, pitch and frequency): ____________________
- Vascular sound (presence or absence of bruit sound): ____________________
- Venous rub over the spleen and liver: ____________________
- Friction rub over the spleen and liver: ____________________

Percussion:

- Percuss for tone (tympani and dull sound at different locations): ____________________
- The span or height of the liver: ____________________
- Spleen: ____________________
- Blunt percussion to find tenderness and muscular resistance: ____________________
- Deep palpation at all 4 quadrants to delineate abdominal organs and detect subtle masses: ____________________
- Assess for masses (in all quadrants): ____________________
- Umbilicus and surroundings: ____________________
- Liver (usually not palpable): ____________________
- Spleen (rarely palpable at left costal margin): ____________________
- Kidney (usually not palpable): ____________________
- Urinary bladder: ____________________

Special Test:

- Ascites (shifting dullness, fluid wave, etc.): ____________________
- Appendicitis (rebound tenderness, psoas sign, obturator sign, hypersensitivity test): ____________________

GAIT

Inspection:

- Patient's ability to walk and move around: ____________________
- Foot position, posture and arm swing during walk: ____________________
- Temporomandibular joint—inspection and palpation: ____________________
- Sternoclavicular joint—inspection and palpation: ____________________
- Cervical, thoracic and lumbar vertebra—inspection and palpation: ____________________

Movement of Cervical Spine:

- Flexion and hyperextension: ______
- Lateral bending: ______
- Rotation: ______

Movement of Thoracic and Lumbar Spine:

- Flexion and extension: ______
- Lateral bending: ______
- Rotation: ______
- Measure leg length: ______
- Straight leg test: ______

SHOULDER AND ARM

Inspection and Palpation:

- Assess for symmetry, color, swelling and masses: ______

Movement:

- Flexion and hyperextension: ______
- Adduction and abduction: ______
- External and internal rotation: ______

ELBOW

Inspection and Palpation:

- Assess size, shape, deformities, redness or swelling: ______

Movement:

- Flexion and extension: ______
- Supination and pronation: ______
- External and pronation: ______

WRIST

Inspection and Palpation:

- Assess size, shape symmetry, color, swelling: ______

- Presence of tenderness and nodules: ______
- Any tenderness in anatomical snuffbox: ______

Movement:

- Flexion and extension: ______
- Radial and ulnar deviation: ______
- Carpal tunnel syndrome: ______
- Phalen's test: ______
- Tinel's test: ______
- Flick test: ______
- Test for thumb weakness: ______

HANDS AND FINGERS

Inspection and Palpation:

- Assess size, shape symmetry, color, swelling: ______
- Palpate for tenderness, swelling bony prominence, nodules or crepitus: ______

Movement:

- Abduction and adduction: ______
- Flexion hyperextension: ______
- Internal and external hip rotation: ______

KNEE

Inspection and Palpation:

- Assess size, shape symmetry, swelling, deformities and alignment: ______
- On palpation knee (tenderness, warmth, consciousness, consistency nodule): ______

Movement:

- Flexion and hyperextension: ______
- Ballottement test: ______
- Mercury test: ______

ANKLES AND FEET

Inspection and Palpation:

- Assess patient in sitting, standing and walking for position, alignment, shape and skin of toe and feet: ____________
- Palpation of ankles and feet (tenderness, heat, swelling or nodule, pain): ____________
- Metatarsophalangeal joint (pain/tenderness): ____________

Movement:

- Dorsiflexion and plantarflexion of foot and ankle: ____________
- Eversion and inversion: ____________
- Abduction and adduction: ____________
- Flexion and extension: ____________

Reflexes:

	Biceps	Triceps	Brachioradialis	Patellar (quadriceps)	Achilles	Ankle clonus
Right side						
Left side						

Superficial Reflexes:

- Abdominal reflex: ____________
- Cremasteric reflex in male patient: ____________
- Test for meningeal irritation: ____________
- Brudziński's sign: ____________
- Kernig's sign: ____________

MALE GENITALIA

Penis

Inspection:

- Urinary catheter (present/absent): ____________________
- Inspect the base part of penis, pubic hairs, skin of the shaft, foreskin, glans: ____________________

Palpation:

- Palpate the shape for tenderness, pain, discharge, etc.____________________

Scrotum

Inspection:

- Inspect the shape, tenderness, and skin scrotum: ____________________

INGUINAL AREA

Inspection:

- Inspect the inguinal femoral areas for any bulge: ____________________

Palpation:

- Palpate on both side of inguinal area for lymph node, masses or bulging, femoral hernia: ____________________

____

FEMALE GENITALIA

External Genitalia

Inspection:

- Urinary catheter (present/absent): ____________________
- Assess the mons pubis, inguinal lymph, labia majora and perineum: ____________________
- Inspect the labia minora, clitoris, urethral meatus and vaginal opening: ____________________

Palpation:

- Bartholin gland (swelling, pain, discharge): ____________________
- Urethra (discharge, tenderness): ____________________

Internal Genitalia

Inspection:

- Observe the size and angle of vaginal opening: ____________________
- Assess vaginal musculature: ____________________
- Inspection of cervix (smoothness, color): ____________________
- Assess the vagina (redness, lesion, color, discharge): ____________________
- Bimanual examination (tenderness, lesion, pain): ____________________

Anus and Rectum

Inspection:

- Insect and opening area for lump, ulcer, lesion, rashes, redness, fissures, thickness of skin: ____________________
- Assess Valsalva maneuver: ____________________
- Assess sacrococcygeal area for swelling, redness, dimpling or hair, etc.: ____________________

Palpation:

- **Anus:** Any sphincter tightness, bleeding, pain, etc.: ____________________
- **Rectum:** Presence of smoothness, tenderness, nodules, irregularities, etc.: ____________________
- **Prostate gland:** (normally nontender and rubbery): ____________________
- Inspect stool, if available: ____________________

EVALUATION PROFORMA PHYSICAL EXAMINATION

Name of the Student: ______________________

Ward/Unit: ______________________

Date of Submission/Presentation: ______________________

Sl. no	Evaluation criteria	Maximum marks	Marks obtained
1.	Introduction and objective	02	
2.	Planning and organization of examination	02	
3.	Accuracy in the examination steps	05	
4.	Identifies the problem and abnormal findings	05	
5.	Rapport with patient	02	
6.	Techniques of question and answer	03	
7.	Recording and reporting	02	
8.	Time management	02	
9.	Conclusion	02	
Total		**25**	

Remarks: ______________________

Signature of the Student

Signature of the Supervisor/Evaluator

PHYSICAL EXAMINATION–2

BIOGRAPHICAL DATA OF PATIENT

Name of the Patient: ____________________ Age: ________ Gender: ____________

Date of Health History Collection: ____________________ Date of Admission: ____________

Hospital/IP No: ____________________ Language Spoken: ____________

Marital Status: ____________ Educational Status: ____________ Religion: ____________

Occupation: ____________________ Provisional Diagnosis: ____________

Treatment under Doctor: ____________________

Name of the procedure (if surgery/procedure done): ____________________

CHIEF COMPLAINTS

HISTORY OF PRESENT ILLNESS

PAST MEDICAL HISTORY

- Past illness and treatment (birth problem/childhood illness/immunization history): History of blood transfusion:
- Any allergic history (food/medication/other):
- Any other relevant (physical/psychological or mental illness):
- Previous hospitalization:

SOCIOECONOMIC STATUS

FAMILY HISTORY OF ANY ILLNESS

Family Tree Diagram:

Genogram Key	
Female	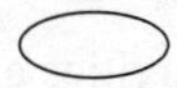
Male	
Patient	
Deceased	 OR 
Cause of death	( )
Adoption (vertical)	|====
Consanguinity	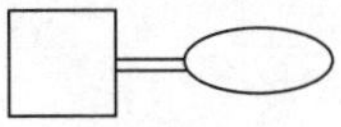

(For reference)

History of chronic illness such as: (diabetes mellitus, hypertension, coronary artery disease, renal disease, psychiatric illness, cancer, etc.): ______

History of any recent death in the family: ______

History of any hereditary disease or communicable disease in the family: ______

PERSONAL HISTORY

- Personal hygiene: ______
- Dietary history (veg/non-veg/meal pattern, any practice): ______

- Elimination pattern: ____________________

- Physical activities and exercises: ____________________

- Work pattern (type, level of job satisfaction, work stress, etc.): ____________________

- Sleeping/rest pattern: ____________________

- Hobbies: ____________________

- Use of any addictive substances: ____________________

- Relationship with patient, friends, significant others: ____________________

- Social activities and religious activities: ____________________

PHYSICAL EXAMINATION

GENERAL APPEARANCE

- **Level of consciousness**: (consciousness/unconsciousness/semi-consciousness/coma/confused, etc.):
 ____
- Orientation (time/place/person): ______________________________
- Mood: ______________________________
- Activity: ______________________________
- Body built: ______________________________

Weight: ____________ **Height** (inches/cm): ____________ **BMI** (weight (kg)/height in meter²): ____________

VITAL SIGNS

Day/Date	Temperature (In °F/°C)	Pulse (beats/min)	Respiration (breaths/min)	Blood pressure (mm Hg)	Pain score on VAS

VISUAL ANALOGUE PAIN (VAS) SCALE

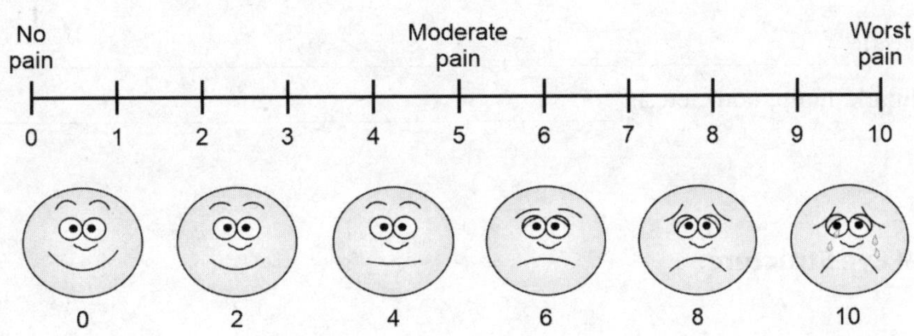

HEAD TO FEET EXAMINATION

HEAD

Inspection and Palpation:

- Hair (distribution/color/clean dry, etc.) ____________________
- Any abrasions/wound/any device: ____________________
- Scalp (clean, dandruff, pediculosis, etc.): ____________________
- Size, shape and configuration: ____________________
- Any involuntary movements: ____________________

FACE

Inspection and Palpation:

- Shape, movement, expression and skin: ____________________
- On palpation of temporal artery: ____________________
- Palpation of temporomandibular joint (TMJ): ____________________

NECK

Inspection:

- Position, symmetry, lump or mass: ____________________
- Movement of neck structure: ____________________
- Cervical vertebrae: ____________________

Palpation:

- Trachea (position/mass): ____________________
- Thyroid gland (landmark, lump, node, etc.): ____________________

EYE (VISION)

Inspection of External Eye Structure:

- Eyelids and eyelashes: ____________________
- Lid margin (ptosis retracted lid margin): ____________________

- Ability to close eyelids: ____________________
- Any redness, swelling, discharge or lesion: ____________________
- Position alignment of the eyeball in the socket: ____________________
- Bulbar conjunctiva and sclera: ____________________
- Cornea and lens: ____________________
- Iris and pupil: ____________________
- Pupillary reaction to light: ____________________

Internal Eye Structure (Use Ophthalmoscope):

- Red reflects (round, regular border/black spots, etc.) ____________________
- Optic disc: ____________________
- Any foreign body, wound laceration, edema: ____________________

EAR (HEARING)

External Ear Structure

Inspection:

- Use of ear hearing aids: ____________________
- Appearance of auricle, tragus, lobule (size/position/color/discharge, etc.): ____________________

Palpation:

- Auricle and mastoids process (pain/tenderness): ____________________

Internal Ear Structure

Inspection:

- Auditory canal (color/earwax/any nodule): ____________________
- Tympanic membrane eardrum (color, shape, consistency, etc.): ____________________

Hearing and Equilibrium Test:

- Whisper test: ____________________
- Weber's test: ____________________
- Rinne test: ____________________
- Romberg test: ____________________

MOUTH, THROAT AND NOSE

Mouth

Inspection and palpation:

- Lips (consistency/color): ____________________
- Teeth (no. of teeth present/color/condition, etc.): ____________________
- Gums (color/consistency/lesion/mass, etc.): ____________________
- Ventral surface of tongue (color/lesion, etc.): ____________________
- Wharton ducts (color, swelling or pain, etc.): ____________________
- Sides of tongue: ____________________
- Strength of tongue: ____________________
- Hard and soft palate and uvula (color/consistency/lesion, etc.): ____________________
- Odor from mouth (any foul odor): ____________________
- Uvula (position/color): ____________________
- Tonsils (color/size/any lesion or exudate, etc.): ____________________
- Posterior pharyngeal wall (color/any lesion or exudate, etc.): ____________________

Throat

Inspection:

- Inspect for nasal flaring and pursed lip breathing: ____________________
- Observe color of face, lips and chest: ____________________
- Inspect color of face, lips and chest: ____________________
- Inspect color and shape of nails: ____________________
- Patient is on: room air/oxygen/BiPAP/ventilator: ____________________
- If no O_2 support: Flow rate: ____________________ Mode: ____________________
- Endotracheal tube (present/absent) size: ____________________
- Respiratory pattern: ____________________

Nose

Inspection:

- External nose: ____________________
- Olfactory sense: ____________________
- Nasal septum: ____________________

POSTERIOR THORAX

Inspection:

- Scapula and spinous process (symmetry, shape, etc.): ______
- Use of accessory muscle (trapezius/shoulder): ______
- Sitting position: ______

Palpation:

- Sensation and tenderness (warm/cold/sensation/pain/lesion/mass, etc.): ______
- Crepitus: ______
- Tactile fremitus (equal bilaterally): ______
- Assess chest expansion: ______

Percussion:

- Tone (resonance/hyperresonance): ______
- Diaphragmatic excursion (normally 3–5 cm): ______

Auscultation:

- Breathing sound heard (normal/abnormal, e.g., crackles/rhonchi/wheezes/pleural friction/rub/stridor/any other, etc.):

  ______

Breathing sound at:

- Vesicular: ______
- Bronchial: ______
- Bronchovesicular: ______
- Adventitious sound (present/absent): ______

ANTERIOR THORAX

Inspection:

- Shape and configuration (symmetry/shape, etc.): ______
- Ratio of anteroposterior verses transverse diameter (normal 1:2): ______
- Position of sternum: ______
- Sternal retraction: ______
- Slope of the ribs: ______
- Quality of accessory muscles (spermatoid/rectus abdominis, etc.): ______

- Intercostal space (retraction/bulging): ___
- Use of accessory muscles (sternomastoid rectus abdominis): ___

Palpation:

- Sensation and tenderness (warm/cold/sensation/lesion/mass, etc.): ___
- Crepitus: ___
- Tactile fremitus (equal bilaterally): ___
- Assess chest expansion: ___

Percussion:

- Tone (resonance/hyperresonance): ___
- Diaphragmatic excursion (normally 3–5 cm): ___

Auscultation:

Breathing sound heard (normal/abnormal—e.g., crackles/rhonchi/wheezes/pleural friction/rub/stridor/any other, etc.):

___

Breathing sound at:

- Vesicular: ___
- Bronchial: ___
- Bronchovesicular: ___
- Adventitious sound (present/absent): ___
- Anterior thorax: ___
- Inspection: ___
- Shape and configuration (system/shape, etc.): ___
- Ratio of anteroposterior verses transverse diameter (normal 1:2): ___
- Position of sternum: ___
- Sternal retraction: ___
- Slope of the ribs: ___
- Quality and pattern of respiration: ___
- Intercostal space: (retraction/bulging): ___
- Use of accessory muscle (sternomastoid/rectus abdominis): ___

Palpation:

- Sensation and tenderness (warm/cold sensation/pain/lesion/mass, etc.): ___

- Crepitus: ____________________
- Tactile fremitus (equal bilaterally): ____________________
- Assess the chest expansion: ____________________

Percussion:

- Tone (resonance/hyperresonance): ____________________
- Diaphragmatic excursion (normally 3–5 cm): ____________________

Auscultation:

- Breathing sound heard (normal/abnormal, crackles/wheezes/pleural friction/rub/stridor/any other, etc.):

____

- Breathing sound at: ____________________
- Vesicular: ____________________
- Bronchial: ____________________
- Bronchovesicular: ____________________
- Adventitious sound (present/absent): ____________________

CHEST INSPECTION

- Size and symmetry: ____________________
- Color and texture: ____________________
- Superficial venous pattern: ____________________
- Areola (color/size/shape/texture): ____________________
- Nipple (size/direction/discharge/lesion, etc.) ____________________
- Retraction or dimpling:

FEMALE BREAST

Palpation:

- Tenderness and temperature: ____________________
- Mass (size/location/shape, etc.): ____________________
- Nipple (discharge): ____________________
- Scar (mastectomy/lumpectomy): ____________________

AXILLA

Inspection and Palpation:

- Mass/tenderness/lesion, etc.: ____________________

MALE BREAST

Areolas, Nipple, and Axilla

Inspection and palpation:

- Any swelling include/nodule/discharge, etc.: ____________________

NECK

Inspection:

- Jugular venous pulses: ____________________

Auscultation and Palpation:

- Auscultate carotid artery (bruit/blowing/swishing sound): ____________________
- Palpate carotid artery (elasticity/thrillers): ____________________

HEART (PERICARDIUM)

Inspection:

- Pulsation (visible location): ____________________

Palpation:

- Apical impulses (present/absent/location): ____________________

Auscultation:

- Rate (per minute): Regular/irregular rhythm: ____________________
- S1 (lub) and S2 (dub) sound: ____________________
- Extra heart sound: ____________________

ARMS

Inspection:

- Color, size, venous pattern and edema: ____________________

Palpation:

- Fingers, hands, arms and warmth: ____________________
- Capillary refill time: ____________________
- Radial pulse (elasticity and strength): ____________________
- Ulnar pulse (present/absent): ____________________
- Brachial pulse (strength): ____________________
- Allen test: ____________________

LEGS

Inspection, Palpation and Auscultation:

- Distribution of hair: ____________________
- Any lesions or ulcer: ____________________
- Edema with characteristics: ____________________
- Varicosities temperature of feet and legs: ____________________
- On palpation of superficial inguinal lymph nodes: ____________________
- On palpation superficial pulse (amplifier and strength): ____________________
- On auscultation of femoral pulse (amplitude and strength): ____________________
- On palpation of popliteal pulse: ____________________
- On palpation of dorsalis pedis pulse (strong/weak/absent): ____________________
- On palpation posterior tibia pulses (strong/weak/absent: ____________________

ABDOMEN

Inspection:

- Color of skin: ____________________
- Vascularity of the skin: ____________________
- Presence of scar: ____________________
- Assess for lesions and rashes: ____________________
- Observe for umbilical for skin color, location and contour: ____________________
- Abdominal contour (flat/rounded/scaphoid): ____________________
- Symmetry: ____________________
- Aortic pulsation: ____________________
- Peristaltic waves: ____________________
- Observable wave: ____________________

Auscultation:

Note: While doing the assessment of abdomen, auscultation is done before percussion and palpation, as their steps may alter the bowel sound.

- Bowel sound (intensity, pitch and frequency): ____________________
- Vascular sound (presence or absence of bruit sound): ____________________
- Venous rub over the spleen and liver: ____________________
- Friction rub over the spleen and liver: ____________________

Percussion:

- Percuss for tone (tympani and dull sound at different locations): ____________________
- The span or height of the liver: ____________________
- Spleen: ____________________
- Blunt percussion to find tenderness and muscular resistance: ____________________
- Deep palpation at all 4 quadrants to delineate abdominal organs and detect subtle masses: ____________________
- Assess for masses (in all quadrants): ____________________
- Umbilicus and surroundings: ____________________
- Liver (usually not palpable): ____________________
- Spleen (rarely palpable at left costal margin): ____________________
- Kidney (usually not palpable): ____________________
- Urinary bladder: ____________________

Special Test:

- Ascites (shifting dullness, fluid wave, etc.) ____________________
- Appendicitis (rebound tenderness, psoas sign, obturator sign, hypersensitivity test): ____________________

GAIT

Inspection:

- Patient's ability to walk and move around: ____________________
- Foot position, posture and arm swing during walk: ____________________
- Temporomandibular joint—inspection and palpation: ____________________
- Sternoclavicular joint—inspection and palpation: ____________________
- Cervical, thoracic and lumbar vertebra—inspection and palpation: ____________________

Movement of Cervical Spine:

- Flexion and hyperextension: ____________________
- Lateral bending: ____________________
- Rotation: ____________________

Movement of Thoracic and Lumbar Spine:

- Flexion and extension: ____________________
- Lateral bending: ____________________
- Rotation: ____________________
- Measure leg length: ____________________
- Straight leg test: ____________________

SHOULDER AND ARM

Inspection and Palpation:

- Assess for symmetry, color, swelling and masses:

Movement:

- Flexion and hyperextension: ____________________
- Adduction and abduction: ____________________
- External and internal rotation: ____________________

ELBOW

Inspection and Palpation:

- Assess size, shape, deformities, redness or swelling: ____________________

Movement:

- Flexion and extension: ____________________
- Supination and pronation: ____________________
- External and pronation: ____________________

WRIST

Inspection and Palpation:

- Assess size, shape symmetry, color, swelling: ____________________

- Presence of tenderness and nodules: ____________________
- Any tenderness in anatomical snuffbox: ____________________

Movement:

- Flexion and extension: ____________________
- Radial and ulnar deviation: ____________________

- Carpal tunnel syndrome: ____________________
- Phalen's test: ____________________
- Tinel's test: ____________________
- Flick test: ____________________
- Test for thumb weakness: ____________________

HANDS AND FINGERS

Inspection and Palpation:

- Assess size, shape symmetry, color, swelling: ____________________
- Palpate for tenderness, swelling bony prominence, nodules or crepitus: ____________________

Movement:

- Abduction and adduction: ____________________
- Flexion hyperextension: ____________________
- Internal and external hip rotation: ____________________

KNEE

Inspection and Palpation:

- Assess size, shape symmetry, swelling, deformities and alignment: ____________________
- On palpation knee (tenderness, warmth, consciousness, consistency nodule): ____________________

Movement:

- Flexion and hyperextension: ____________________
- Ballottement test: ____________________
- Mercury test: ____________________

ANKLES AND FEET

Inspection and Palpation:

- Assess patient in sitting, standing and walking for position, alignment, shape and skin of toe and feet: ____________
- Palpation of ankles and feet (tenderness, heat, swelling or nodule, pain): ____________
- Metatarsophalangeal joint (pain/tenderness): ____________

Movement:

- Dorsiflexion and plantarflexion of foot and ankle: ____________
- Eversion and inversion: ____________
- Abduction and adduction: ____________
- Flexion and extension: ____________

Reflexes:

	Biceps	Triceps	Brachioradialis	Patellar (quadriceps)	Achilles	Ankle clonus
Right side						
Left side						

Superficial Reflexes:

- Abdominal reflex: ____________
- Cremasteric reflex in male patient: ____________
- Test for meningeal irritation: ____________
- Brudziński's sign: ____________
- Kernig's sign: ____________

MALE GENITALIA

Penis

Inspection:

- Urinary catheter (present/absent): ____________________
- Inspect the base part of penis, pubic hairs, skin of the shaft, foreskin, glans: ____________________

Palpation:

- Palpate the shape for tenderness, pain, discharge, etc.____________________

Scrotum

Inspection:

- Inspect the shape, tenderness, and skin scrotum: ____________________

INGUINAL AREA

Inspection:

- Inspect the inguinal femoral areas for any bulge: ____________________

Palpation:

- Palpate on both side of inguinal area for lymph node, masses or bulging, femoral hernia: ____________________

____

FEMALE GENITALIA

External Genitalia

Inspection:

- Urinary catheter (present/absent): ____________________
- Assess the mons pubis, inguinal lymph, labia majora and perineum: ____________________
- Inspect the labia minora, clitoris, urethral meatus and vaginal opening: ____________________

Palpation:

- Bartholin gland (swelling, pain, discharge): ____________________
- Urethra (discharge, tenderness): ____________________

Internal Genitalia

Inspection:

- Observe the size and angle of vaginal opening: ______
- Assess vaginal musculature: ______
- Inspection of cervix (smoothness, color): ______
- Assess the vagina (redness, lesion, color, discharge): ______
- Bimanual examination (tenderness, lesion, pain): ______

Anus and Rectum

Inspection:

- Insect and opening area for lump, ulcer, lesion, rashes, redness, fissures, thickness of skin: ______
- Assess Valsalva maneuver: ______
- Assess sacrococcygeal area for swelling, redness, dimpling or hair, etc.: ______

Palpation:

- **Anus:** Any sphincter tightness, bleeding, pain, etc. ______
- **Rectum:** Presence of smoothness, tenderness, nodules, irregularities, etc.: ______
- **Prostate gland:** (normally nontender and rubbery): ______
- Inspect stool, if available: ______

EVALUATION PROFORMA PHYSICAL EXAMINATION

Name of the Student: ____________________

Ward/Unit: ____________________

Date of Submission/Presentation: ____________________

Sl. no	Evaluation criteria	Maximum marks	Marks obtained
1.	Introduction and objective	02	
2.	Planning and organization of examination	02	
3.	Accuracy in the examination steps	05	
4.	Identifies the problem and abnormal findings	05	
5.	Rapport with patient	02	
6.	Techniques of question and answer	03	
7.	Recording and reporting	02	
8.	Time management	02	
9.	Conclusion	02	
Total		**25**	

Remarks: ____________________

Signature of the Student

Signature of the Supervisor/Evaluator

CLINICAL EXPERIENCE DETAILS

Name of the clinical areas	Clinical condition	Number of days care given	Signature of Faculty/Preceptor

Signature of the Faculty Coordinator

Signature of the HOD/Principal

Signature of the Internal Examiner

Name: ______________________

Date: ______________________

Signature of the External Examiner

Name: ______________________

Date: ______________________

Supplementary Examination:

Signature of the Internal Examiner

Name: ______________________

Date: ______________________

Signature of the External Examiner

Name: ______________________

Date: ______________________

Semester II

NURSING PROCESS–1

BIOGRAPHICAL DATA OF PATIENT

Name of the Patient: ______________________ Age: ________ Gender: ____________

Date of Health History Collection: ____________________ Date of Admission: ______________

Hospital/IP No: ____________________ Language Spoken: ______________________

Marital Status: ____________ Educational Status: ____________ Religion: ____________

Occupation: ____________________ Provisional Diagnosis: ______________________

Treatment under Doctor: ____

Name of the procedure (if surgery/procedure done): ______________________________

CHIEF COMPLAINTS

HISTORY OF PRESENT ILLNESS

PAST MEDICAL HISTORY

- Past illness and treatment (birth problem/childhood illness/immunization history): History of blood transfusion:

- Any allergic history (food/medication/other):

- Any other relevant (physical/psychological or mental illness):

- Previous hospitalization:

SOCIOECONOMIC STATUS

FAMILY HISTORY OF ANY ILLNESS

Family Tree Diagram:

Genogram Key	
Female	○
Male	□
Patient	↗
Deceased	■ OR ●
Cause of death	( )
Adoption (vertical)	|====
Consanguinity	□=○

(For reference)

History of chronic illness such as: (diabetes mellitus, hypertension, coronary artery disease, renal disease, psychiatric illness, cancer, etc.): ____________________

____

____

History of any recent death in the family: ____________________

____

____

History of any hereditary disease or communicable disease in the family: ____________________

____

PERSONAL HISTORY

- Personal hygiene: ____________________

  ____

- Dietary history (veg/non-veg/meal pattern, any practice): ____________________

  ____

- Elimination pattern: ____________________
- Physical activities and exercises: ____________________
- Work pattern (type, level of job satisfaction, work stress, etc.): ____________________
- Sleeping/rest pattern: ____________________
- Hobbies: ____________________
- Use of any addictive substances: ____________________
- Relationship with patient, friends, significant others: ____________________
- Social activities and religious activities: ____________________

PHYSICAL EXAMINATION

GENERAL APPEARANCE

- **Level of consciousness**: (consciousness/unconsciousness/semi-consciousness/coma/confused, etc.): ______________________________
- Orientation (time/place/person): ______________________________
- Mood: ______________________________
- Activity: ______________________________
- Body built: ______________________________

Weight: ____________ **Height** (inches/cm): ____________ **BMI** (weight (kg)/height in meter^2): ____________

VITAL SIGNS

Day/Date	Temperature (In °F/°C)	Pulse (beats/min)	Respiration (breaths/min)	Blood pressure (mm Hg)	Pain score on VAS

VISUAL ANALOGUE PAIN (VAS) SCALE

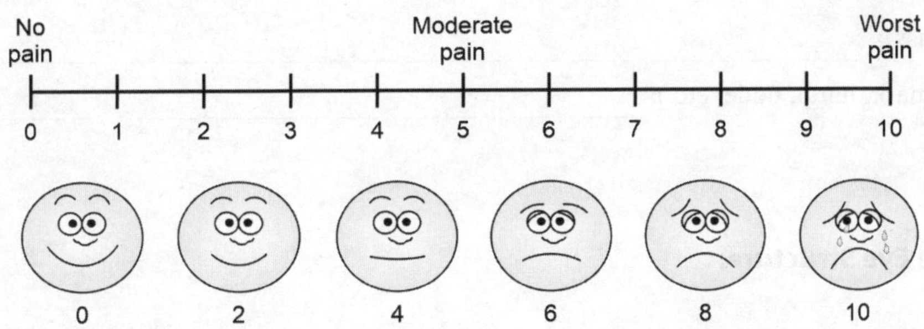

HEAD TO FEET EXAMINATION

HEAD

Inspection and Palpation:

- Hair (distribution/color/clean dry, etc.) ____________________
- Any abrasions/wound/any device: ____________________
- Scalp (clean, dandruff, pediculosis, etc.): ____________________
- Size, shape and configuration: ____________________
- Any involuntary movements: ____________________

FACE

Inspection and Palpation:

- Shape, movement, expression and skin: ____________________
- On palpation of temporal artery: ____________________
- Palpation of temporomandibular joint (TMJ): ____________________

NECK

Inspection:

- Position, symmetry, lump or mass: ____________________
- Movement of neck structure: ____________________
- Cervical vertebrae: ____________________

Palpation:

- Trachea (position/mass): ____________________
- Thyroid gland (landmark, lump, node, etc.): ____________________

EYE (VISION)

Inspection of External Eye Structure:

- Eyelids and eyelashes: ____________________
- Lid margin (ptosis retracted lid margin): ____________________

- Ability to close eyelids: ______
- Any redness, swelling, discharge or lesion: ______
- Position alignment of the eyeball in the socket: ______
- Bulbar conjunctiva and sclera: ______
- Cornea and lens: ______
- Iris and pupil: ______
- Pupillary reaction to light: ______

Internal Eye Structure (Use Ophthalmoscope):

- Red reflects (round, regular border/black spots, etc.) ______
- Optic disc: ______
- Any foreign body, wound laceration, edema: ______

EAR (HEARING)

External Ear Structure

Inspection:

- Use of ear hearing aids: ______
- Appearance of auricle, tragus, lobule (size/position/color/discharge, etc.): ______

Palpation:

- Auricle and mastoids process (pain/tenderness): ______

Internal Ear Structure

Inspection:

- Auditory canal (color/earwax/any nodule): ______
- Tympanic membrane eardrum (color, shape, consistency, etc.): ______

Hearing and Equilibrium Test:

- Whisper test: ______
- Weber's test: ______
- Rinne test: ______
- Romberg test: ______

MOUTH, THROAT AND NOSE

Mouth

Inspection and palpation:

- Lips (consistency/color): ______
- Teeth (no. of teeth present/color/condition, etc.): ______
- Gums (color/consistency/lesion/mass, etc.): ______
- Ventral surface of tongue (color/lesion, etc.): ______
- Wharton ducts (color, swelling or pain, etc.): ______
- Sides of tongue: ______
- Strength of tongue: ______
- Hard and soft palate and uvula (color/consistency/lesion, etc.): ______
- Odor from mouth (any foul odor): ______
- Uvula (position/color): ______
- Tonsils (color/size/any lesion or exudate, etc.): ______
- Posterior pharyngeal wall (color/any lesion or exudate, etc.): ______

Throat

Inspection:

- Inspect for nasal flaring and pursed lip breathing: ______
- Observe color of face, lips and chest: ______
- Inspect color of face, lips and chest: ______
- Inspect color and shape of nails: ______
- Patient is on: room air/oxygen/BiPAP/ventilator: ______
- If no O_2 support: Flow rate: ______ Mode: ______
- Endotracheal tube (present/absent) size: ______
- Respiratory pattern: ______

Nose

Inspection:

- External nose: ______
- Olfactory sense: ______
- Nasal septum: ______

POSTERIOR THORAX

Inspection:

- Scapula and spinous process (symmetry, shape, etc.): ____________________
- Use of accessory muscle (trapezius/shoulder): ____________________
- Sitting position: ____________________

Palpation:

- Sensation and tenderness (warm/cold/sensation/pain/lesion/mass, etc.): ____________________
- Crepitus: ____________________
- Tactile fremitus (equal bilaterally): ____________________
- Assess chest expansion: ____________________

Percussion:

- Tone (resonance/hyperresonance): ____________________
- Diaphragmatic excursion (normally 3–5 cm): ____________________

Auscultation:

- Breathing sound heard (normal/abnormal, e.g., crackles/rhonchi/wheezes/pleural friction/rub/stridor/any other, etc.):

  ____

Breathing sound at:

- Vesicular: ____________________
- Bronchial: ____________________
- Bronchovesicular: ____________________
- Adventitious sound (present/absent): ____________________

ANTERIOR THORAX

Inspection:

- Shape and configuration (symmetry/shape, etc.): ____________________
- Ratio of anteroposterior verses transverse diameter (normal 1:2): ____________________
- Position of sternum: ____________________
- Sternal retraction: ____________________
- Slope of the ribs: ____________________
- Quality of accessory muscles (spermatoid/rectus abdominis, etc.): ____________________

- Intercostal space (retraction/bulging): ____________________
- Use of accessory muscles (sternomastoid rectus abdominis): ____________________

Palpation:

- Sensation and tenderness (warm/cold/sensation/lesion/mass, etc.): ____________________
- Crepitus: ____________________
- Tactile fremitus (equal bilaterally): ____________________
- Assess chest expansion: ____________________

Percussion:

- Tone (resonance/hyperresonance): ____________________
- Diaphragmatic excursion (normally 3–5 cm): ____________________

Auscultation:

Breathing sound heard (normal/abnormal—e.g., crackles/rhonchi/wheezes/pleural friction/rub/stridor/any other, etc.):

____

Breathing sound at:

- Vesicular: ____________________
- Bronchial: ____________________
- Bronchovesicular: ____________________
- Adventitious sound (present/absent): ____________________
- Anterior thorax: ____________________
- Inspection: ____________________
- Shape and configuration (system/shape, etc.): ____________________
- Ratio of anteroposterior verses transverse diameter (normal 1:2): ____________________
- Position of sternum: ____________________
- Sternal retraction: ____________________
- Slope of the ribs: ____________________
- Quality and pattern of respiration: ____________________
- Intercostal space: (retraction/bulging): ____________________
- Use of accessory muscle (sternomastoid/rectus abdominis): ____________________

Palpation:

- Sensation and tenderness (warm/cold sensation/pain/lesion/mass, etc.): ____________________

- Crepitus: ____________________
- Tactile fremitus (equal bilaterally): ____________________
- Assess the chest expansion: ____________________

Percussion:

- Tone (resonance/hyperresonance): ____________________
- Diaphragmatic excursion (normally 3–5 cm): ____________________

Auscultation:

- Breathing sound heard (normal/abnormal, crackles/wheezes/pleural friction/rub/stridor/any other, etc.):
  ____
- Breathing sound at: ____________________
- Vesicular: ____________________
- Bronchial: ____________________
- Bronchovesicular: ____________________
- Adventitious sound (present/absent): ____________________

CHEST INSPECTION

- Size and symmetry: ____________________
- Color and texture: ____________________
- Superficial venous pattern: ____________________
- Areola (color/size/shape/texture): ____________________
- Nipple (size/direction/discharge/lesion, etc.) ____________________
- Retraction or dimpling:

FEMALE BREAST

Palpation:

- Tenderness and temperature: ____________________
- Mass (size/location/shape, etc.): ____________________
- Nipple (discharge): ____________________
- Scar (mastectomy/lumpectomy): ____________________

AXILLA

Inspection and Palpation:

- Mass/tenderness/lesion, etc.: ____________________

MALE BREAST

Areolas, Nipple, and Axilla

Inspection and palpation:

- Any swelling include/nodule/discharge, etc.: ____________________

NECK

Inspection:

- Jugular venous pulses: ____________________

Auscultation and Palpation:

- Auscultate carotid artery (bruit/blowing/swishing sound): ____________________
- Palpate carotid artery (elasticity/thrillers): ____________________

HEART (PERICARDIUM)

Inspection:

- Pulsation (visible location): ____________________

Palpation:

- Apical impulses (present/absent/location): ____________________

Auscultation:

- Rate (per minute): Regular/irregular rhythm: ____________________
- S1 (lub) and S2 (dub) sound: ____________________
- Extra heart sound: ____________________

ARMS

Inspection:

- Color, size, venous pattern and edema: ____________________

Palpation:

- Fingers, hands, arms and warmth: ______
- Capillary refill time: ______
- Radial pulse (elasticity and strength): ______
- Ulnar pulse (present/absent): ______
- Brachial pulse (strength): ______
- Allen test: ______

LEGS

Inspection, Palpation and Auscultation:

- Distribution of hair: ______
- Any lesions or ulcer: ______
- Edema with characteristics: ______
- Varicosities temperature of feet and legs: ______
- On palpation of superficial inguinal lymph nodes: ______
- On palpation superficial pulse (amplifier and strength): ______
- On auscultation of femoral pulse (amplitude and strength): ______
- On palpation of popliteal pulse: ______
- On palpation of dorsalis pedis pulse (strong/weak/absent): ______
- On palpation posterior tibia pulses (strong/weak/absent: ______

ABDOMEN

Inspection:

- Color of skin: ______
- Vascularity of the skin: ______
- Presence of scar: ______
- Assess for lesions and rashes: ______
- Observe for umbilical for skin color, location and contour: ______
- Abdominal contour (flat/rounded/scaphoid): ______
- Symmetry: ______
- Aortic pulsation: ______
- Peristaltic waves: ______
- Observable wave: ______

Auscultation:

Note: While doing the assessment of abdomen, auscultation is done before percussion and palpation, as their steps may alter the bowel sound.

- Bowel sound (intensity, pitch and frequency): ________________
- Vascular sound (presence or absence of bruit sound): ________________
- Venous rub over the spleen and liver: ________________
- Friction rub over the spleen and liver: ________________

Percussion:

- Percuss for tone (tympani and dull sound at different locations): ________________
- The span or height of the liver: ________________
- Spleen: ________________
- Blunt percussion to find tenderness and muscular resistance: ________________
- Deep palpation at all 4 quadrants to delineate abdominal organs and detect subtle masses: ________________
- Assess for masses (in all quadrants): ________________
- Umbilicus and surroundings: ________________
- Liver (usually not palpable): ________________
- Spleen (rarely palpable at left costal margin): ________________
- Kidney (usually not palpable): ________________
- Urinary bladder: ________________

Special Test:

- Ascites (shifting dullness, fluid wave, etc.): ________________
- Appendicitis (rebound tenderness, psoas sign, obturator sign, hypersensitivity test): ________________

GAIT

Inspection:

- Patient's ability to walk and move around: ________________
- Foot position, posture and arm swing during walk: ________________
- Temporomandibular joint—inspection and palpation: ________________
- Sternoclavicular joint—inspection and palpation: ________________
- Cervical, thoracic and lumbar vertebra—inspection and palpation: ________________

Movement of Cervical Spine:

- Flexion and hyperextension: ______________________________
- Lateral bending: ______________________________
- Rotation: ______________________________

Movement of Thoracic and Lumbar Spine:

- Flexion and extension: ______________________________
- Lateral bending: ______________________________
- Rotation: ______________________________
- Measure leg length: ______________________________
- Straight leg test: ______________________________

SHOULDER AND ARM

Inspection and Palpation:

- Assess for symmetry, color, swelling and masses: ______________________________

Movement:

- Flexion and hyperextension: ______________________________
- Adduction and abduction: ______________________________
- External and internal rotation: ______________________________

ELBOW

Inspection and Palpation:

- Assess size, shape, deformities, redness or swelling: ______________________________

Movement:

- Flexion and extension: ______________________________
- Supination and pronation: ______________________________
- External and pronation: ______________________________

WRIST

Inspection and Palpation:

- Assess size, shape symmetry, color, swelling: ______________________________

- Presence of tenderness and nodules: ____________________
- Any tenderness in anatomical snuffbox: ____________________

Movement:

  - Flexion and extension: ____________________
  - Radial and ulnar deviation: ____________________

- Carpal tunnel syndrome: ____________________
- Phalen's test: ____________________
- Tinel's test: ____________________
- Flick test: ____________________
- Test for thumb weakness: ____________________

HANDS AND FINGERS

Inspection and Palpation:

- Assess size, shape symmetry, color, swelling: ____________________
- Palpate for tenderness, swelling bony prominence, nodules or crepitus: ____________________

Movement:

- Abduction and adduction: ____________________
- Flexion hyperextension: ____________________
- Internal and external hip rotation: ____________________

KNEE

Inspection and Palpation:

- Assess size, shape symmetry, swelling, deformities and alignment: ____________________
- On palpation knee (tenderness, warmth, consciousness, consistency nodule): ____________________

Movement:

- Flexion and hyperextension: ____________________
- Ballottement test: ____________________
- Mercury test: ____________________

ANKLES AND FEET

Inspection and Palpation:

- Assess patient in sitting, standing and walking for position, alignment, shape and skin of toe and feet: ____________
- Palpation of ankles and feet (tenderness, heat, swelling or nodule, pain): ____________
- Metatarsophalangeal joint (pain/tenderness): ____________

Movement:

- Dorsiflexion and plantarflexion of foot and ankle: ____________
- Eversion and inversion: ____________
- Abduction and adduction: ____________
- Flexion and extension: ____________

Reflexes:

	Biceps	Triceps	Brachioradialis	Patellar (quadriceps)	Achilles	Ankle clonus
Right side						
Left side						

Superficial Reflexes:

- Abdominal reflex: ____________
- Cremasteric reflex in male patient: ____________
- Test for meningeal irritation: ____________
- Brudziński's sign: ____________
- Kernig's sign: ____________

MALE GENITALIA

Penis

Inspection:

- Urinary catheter (present/absent): ____________________
- Inspect the base part of penis, pubic hairs, skin of the shaft, foreskin, glans: ____________________

Palpation:

- Palpate the shape for tenderness, pain, discharge, etc.____________________

Scrotum

Inspection:

- Inspect the shape, tenderness, and skin scrotum: ____________________

INGUINAL AREA

Inspection:

- Inspect the inguinal femoral areas for any bulge: ____________________

Palpation:

- Palpate on both side of inguinal area for lymph node, masses or bulging, femoral hernia: ____________________

____

FEMALE GENITALIA

External Genitalia

Inspection:

- Urinary catheter (present/absent): ____________________
- Assess the mons pubis, inguinal lymph, labia majora and perineum: ____________________
- Inspect the labia minora, clitoris, urethral meatus and vaginal opening: ____________________

Palpation:

- Bartholin gland (swelling, pain, discharge): ____________________
- Urethra (discharge, tenderness): ____________________

Internal Genitalia

Inspection:

- Observe the size and angle of vaginal opening: ________________
- Assess vaginal musculature: ________________
- Inspection of cervix (smoothness, color): ________________
- Assess the vagina (redness, lesion, color, discharge): ________________
- Bimanual examination (tenderness, lesion, pain): ________________

Anus and Rectum

Inspection:

- Insect and opening area for lump, ulcer, lesion, rashes, redness, fissures, thickness of skin: ________________
- Assess Valsalva maneuver: ________________
- Assess sacrococcygeal area for swelling, redness, dimpling or hair, etc.: ________________

Palpation:

- **Anus:** Any sphincter tightness, bleeding, pain, etc. ________________
- **Rectum:** Presence of smoothness, tenderness, nodules, irregularities, etc.: ________________
- **Prostate gland:** (normally nontender and rubbery): ________________
- Inspect stool, if available: ________________

INVESTIGATIONS

BLOOD/PATHOLOGICAL INVESTIGATIONS

Investigations	Normal values	Patient investigations values			Remark
		Date	Date	Date	
HEMATOLOGY					
Hemoglobin	12.5–17.5 g/dL				
RBC	4.50–6.0 × 10^6/mL				
PCV	35.0–50.4%				
MCV	80.0–99.9 fl				
MCH	27.0–31.0 pg.				
MCHC	33.0–37.0 g/dL				
Total WBC	4000–11000/cumm				
DLC: Polymorphs	40–75%				
Lymphocytes	20–40%				
Eosinophil	01–06%				
Monocytes	02–08%				
Basophil	00–01%				
Malaria parasite					
Smear: Normal					
Platelet count	1.5–4.5 lakhs/cumm				
ESR	Up to 15 mm at 1 hour				
AEC	40–440/cumm				
Retic count	0.5–2.5%				
Prothrombin time					
INR					
PTTK					
Bleeding time	1–5 minutes				
Clotting time	3–8 minutes				
Urine: Appearance					
Reaction					
Albumin					

Investigations	Normal values	Patient investigations values			Remark
		Date	Date	Date	
Sugar					
Acetone					
Bile salt/pigments					
Pus cells					
RBCs					
Others					
SEROLOGY: HIV					
HBsAg					
BIOCHEMISTRY					
Blood sugar fasting	70–110 mg/dL				
Postprandial	90–160 mg/dL				
Random	90–160 mg/dL				
HbA1c	4.2–6.2 mg/dL				
Blood urea	14–50 mg/dL				
Serum creatinine	0.6–1.4 mg/dL				
Uric acid	M: 2.7–7.7 mg/dL F: 2.4–5.7 mg/dL				
CPK	Up to 190 IU/L				
CPK MB	Up to 40 IU /L				
SGOT	Up to 40 IU/L				
LDH	Up to 450 IU /L				
Serum sodium	134–148 mEq /L				
Serum potassium	3.5–5.6 mEq/L				
Serum calcium	8.1–10.4 mg/dL				
Serum phosphorous	2.5–4.5 mg/dL				
Serum magnesium	1.8–2.6 mg/dL				
LIPID: Total cholesterol	Up to 200 mg/dL				
HDL cholesterol	40–60 mg/dL				
Serum triglycerides	Up to 150 mg/dL				
LDL cholesterol	Up to 100 mg/dL				

Investigations	Normal values	Patient investigations values			Remark
		Date	Date	Date	
LFT: Total protein	6.0–7.8 g/dL				
Albumin	3.2–4.5 g/dL				
Globulin	2.3–3.5 g/dL				
Bilirubin total	Up to 1.2 mg/dL				
Bilirubin direct	Up to 0.25 mg/dL				
SGPT	Up to 40 IU/L				
Alkaline phosphates	Up to 150 IU/L				
Serum digoxin	0.8–2.0 ng/mL				
Serum amylase	25–125 U/L				
SEROLOGY					
RA:					
CRP:					
ASO:					
TROP- T					

OTHER DIAGNOSTIC INVESTIGATIONS:

Ultrasonography (USG): (abdomen/pelvis/kidney/urethra/bladder (kub) etc.):

____

X-ray: (abdomen/pelvis/kidney/urethra/bladder (KUB) etc.):

____

Computer tomography (CT scan):

____

Magnetic resonance imagination: (MRI):

____

Any other:

____

MEDICATION

Sl. no.	Name of medication, route, dose	Action	Indication	Contraindication	Side effects	Nurses responsibility

LIST OF NURSING DIAGNOSIS ACCORDING TO PRIORITY

NURSING CARE PLAN

Assessment	Nursing diagnosis	Expected outcome	Planning intervention	Rationale	Evaluation
Subjective data:		**Short-term outcome:**			
Objective data:		**Long-term outcome:**			

NURSING CARE PLAN

Assessment	Nursing diagnosis	Expected outcome	Planning intervention	Rationale	Evaluation
Subjective data:		**Short-term outcome:**			
Objective data:		**Long-term outcome:**			

NURSING CARE PLAN

Assessment	Nursing diagnosis	Expected outcome	Planning intervention	Rationale	Evaluation
Subjective data: **Objective data:**		**Short-term outcome:** **Long-term outcome:**			

NURSING CARE PLAN

Assessment	Nursing diagnosis	Expected outcome	Planning intervention	Rationale	Evaluation
Subjective data:		**Short-term outcome:**			
Objective data:		**Long-term outcome:**			

HEALTH EDUCATION

Disease condition: ______________________________

____

____

____

Diet: ______________________________

____

____

____

Personal hygiene: ______________________________

____

____

____

Medication: ______________________________

____

____

____

Lifestyle modification: ______________________________

____

____

____

Follow-up care: ______________________________

____

____

____

BIBLIOGRAPHY/REFERENCES

(Write bibliography in the Vancouver style)

EVALUATION PROFORMA NURSING PROCESS

Name of the Student: ______________________ **Date:** ______________

Clinical Area: ______________________ **Diagnosis:** ______________

Sl. no.	Criteria	Allotted marks	Obtained marks
1.	History collection	3	
2.	Physical examination	3	
3.	Drug study	2	
4.	Nursing assessment	2	
5.	Prioritize the nursing diagnosis	5	
6.	Nursing care plan on 5 need-based nursing diagnosis	5	
7.	Prognosis of patient	1	
8.	Nurses notes	2	
9.	Bibliography/References	2	
Total		**25**	

Remarks: ______________________________

Signature of the Student **Signature of the Evaluator**

NURSING PROCESS–2

BIOGRAPHICAL DATA OF PATIENT

Name of the Patient: ______________________ Age: __________ Gender: ______________

Date of Health History Collection: ______________________ Date of Admission: ______________

Hospital/IP No: ______________________ Language Spoken: ______________________

Marital Status: ______________ Educational Status: ______________ Religion: ______________

Occupation: ______________________ Provisional Diagnosis: ______________________

Treatment under Doctor: ____

Name of the procedure (if surgery/procedure done): ______________________________

CHIEF COMPLAINTS

____

____

____

____

____

HISTORY OF PRESENT ILLNESS

____

____

____

____

____

PAST MEDICAL HISTORY

- Past illness and treatment (birth problem/childhood illness/immunization history): History of blood transfusion: ____________________
- Any allergic history (food/medication/other): ____________________
- Any other relevant (physical/psychological or mental illness): ____________________
- Previous hospitalization: ____________________

SOCIOECONOMIC STATUS

____

FAMILY HISTORY OF ANY ILLNESS

____

Family Tree Diagram:

Genogram Key	
Female	⬭
Male	□
Patient	↗
Deceased	■ OR ⬬
Cause of death	( )
Adoption (vertical)	|====
Consanguinity	□═⬭

(For reference)

History of chronic illness such as: (diabetes mellitus, hypertension, coronary artery disease, renal disease, psychiatric illness, cancer, etc.): ______________________________

____

____

History of any recent death in the family: ______________________________

____

____

History of any hereditary disease or communicable disease in the family: ______________________________

____

PERSONAL HISTORY

- Personal hygiene: ______________________________

  ____

- Dietary history (veg/non-veg/meal pattern, any practice): ______________________________

  ____

- Elimination pattern: ______________________________

  ____

- Physical activities and exercises: ______________________________

  ____

- Work pattern (type, level of job satisfaction, work stress, etc.): ______________________________

  ____

- Sleeping/rest pattern: ______________________________

  ____

- Hobbies: ______________________________

  ____

- Use of any addictive substances: ______________________________

  ____

- Relationship with patient, friends, significant others: ______________________________

  ____

- Social activities and religious activities: ______________________________

  ____

PHYSICAL EXAMINATION

GENERAL APPEARANCE

- **Level of consciousness**: (consciousness/unconsciousness/semi-consciousness/coma/confused, etc.): ____________________
- Orientation (time/place/person): ____________________
- Mood: ____________________
- Activity: ____________________
- Body built: ____________________

Weight: __________ **Height** (inches/cm): __________ **BMI** (weight (kg)/height in meter^2): __________

VITAL SIGNS

Day/Date	Temperature (In °F/°C)	Pulse (beats/min)	Respiration (breaths/min)	Blood pressure (mm Hg)	Pain score on VAS

VISUAL ANALOGUE PAIN (VAS) SCALE

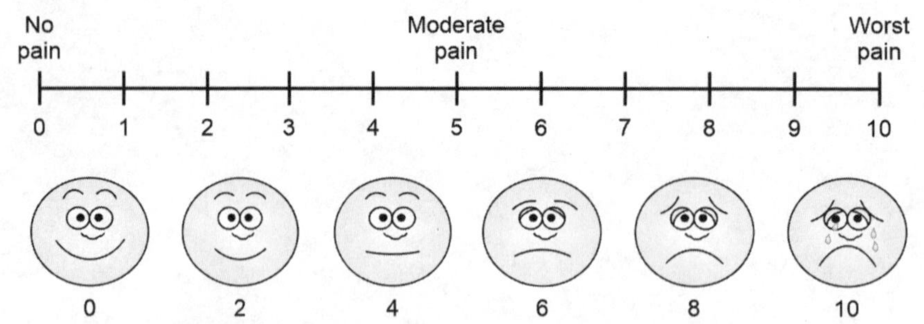

HEAD TO FEET EXAMINATION

HEAD

Inspection and Palpation:

- Hair (distribution/color/clean dry, etc.) ____________________
- Any abrasions/wound/any device: ____________________
- Scalp (clean, dandruff, pediculosis, etc.): ____________________
- Size, shape and configuration: ____________________
- Any involuntary movements: ____________________

FACE

Inspection and Palpation:

- Shape, movement, expression and skin: ____________________
- On palpation of temporal artery: ____________________
- Palpation of temporomandibular joint (TMJ): ____________________

NECK

Inspection:

- Position, symmetry, lump or mass: ____________________
- Movement of neck structure: ____________________
- Cervical vertebrae: ____________________

Palpation:

- Trachea (position/mass): ____________________
- Thyroid gland (landmark, lump, node, etc.): ____________________

EYE (VISION)

Inspection of External Eye Structure:

- Eyelids and eyelashes: ____________________
- Lid margin (ptosis retracted lid margin): ____________________

- Ability to close eyelids: ____________________
- Any redness, swelling, discharge or lesion: ____________________
- Position alignment of the eyeball in the socket: ____________________
- Bulbar conjunctiva and sclera: ____________________
- Cornea and lens: ____________________
- Iris and pupil: ____________________
- Pupillary reaction to light: ____________________

Internal Eye Structure (Use Ophthalmoscope):

- Red reflects (round, regular border/black spots, etc.) ____________________
- Optic disc: ____________________
- Any foreign body, wound laceration, edema: ____________________

EAR (HEARING)

External Ear Structure

Inspection:

- Use of ear hearing aids: ____________________
- Appearance of auricle, tragus, lobule (size/position/color/discharge, etc.): ____________________

Palpation:

- Auricle and mastoids process (pain/tenderness): ____________________

Internal Ear Structure

Inspection:

- Auditory canal (color/earwax/any nodule): ____________________
- Tympanic membrane eardrum (color, shape, consistency, etc.): ____________________

Hearing and Equilibrium Test:

- Whisper test: ____________________
- Weber's test: ____________________
- Rinne test: ____________________
- Romberg test: ____________________

MOUTH, THROAT AND NOSE

Mouth

Inspection and palpation:

- Lips (consistency/color): ______
- Teeth (no. of teeth present/color/condition, etc.): ______
- Gums (color/consistency/lesion/mass, etc.): ______
- Ventral surface of tongue (color/lesion, etc.): ______
- Wharton ducts (color, swelling or pain, etc.): ______
- Sides of tongue: ______
- Strength of tongue: ______
- Hard and soft palate and uvula (color/consistency/lesion, etc.): ______
- Odor from mouth (any foul odor): ______
- Uvula (position/color): ______
- Tonsils (color/size/any lesion or exudate, etc.): ______
- Posterior pharyngeal wall (color/any lesion or exudate, etc.): ______

Throat

Inspection:

- Inspect for nasal flaring and pursed lip breathing: ______
- Observe color of face, lips and chest: ______
- Inspect color of face, lips and chest: ______
- Inspect color and shape of nails: ______
- Patient is on: room air/oxygen/BiPAP/ventilator: ______
- If no O_2 support: Flow rate: ______ Mode: ______
- Endotracheal tube (present/absent) size: ______
- Respiratory pattern: ______

Nose

Inspection:

- External nose: ______
- Olfactory sense: ______
- Nasal septum: ______

POSTERIOR THORAX

Inspection:

- Scapula and spinous process (symmetry, shape, etc.): __________
- Use of accessory muscle (trapezius/shoulder): __________
- Sitting position: __________

Palpation:

- Sensation and tenderness (warm/cold/sensation/pain/lesion/mass, etc.): __________
- Crepitus: __________
- Tactile fremitus (equal bilaterally): __________
- Assess chest expansion: __________

Percussion:

- Tone (resonance/hyperresonance): __________
- Diaphragmatic excursion (normally 3–5 cm): __________

Auscultation:

- Breathing sound heard (normal/abnormal, e.g., crackles/rhonchi/wheezes/pleural friction/rub/stridor/any other, etc.):

  ____

Breathing sound at:

- Vesicular: __________
- Bronchial: __________
- Bronchovesicular: __________
- Adventitious sound (present/absent): __________

ANTERIOR THORAX

Inspection:

- Shape and configuration (symmetry/shape, etc.): __________
- Ratio of anteroposterior verses transverse diameter (normal 1:2): __________
- Position of sternum: __________
- Sternal retraction: __________
- Slope of the ribs: __________
- Quality of accessory muscles (spermatoid/rectus abdominis, etc.): __________

- Intercostal space (retraction/bulging): ____________________
- Use of accessory muscles (sternomastoid rectus abdominis): ____________________

Palpation:

- Sensation and tenderness (warm/cold/sensation/lesion/mass, etc.): ____________________
- Crepitus: ____________________
- Tactile fremitus (equal bilaterally): ____________________
- Assess chest expansion: ____________________

Percussion:

- Tone (resonance/hyperresonance): ____________________
- Diaphragmatic excursion (normally 3–5 cm): ____________________

Auscultation:

Breathing sound heard (normal/abnormal—e.g., crackles/rhonchi/wheezes/pleural friction/rub/stridor/any other, etc.):

____

Breathing sound at:

- Vesicular: ____________________
- Bronchial: ____________________
- Bronchovesicular: ____________________
- Adventitious sound (present/absent): ____________________
- Anterior thorax: ____________________
- Inspection: ____________________
- Shape and configuration (system/shape, etc.): ____________________
- Ratio of anteroposterior verses transverse diameter (normal 1:2): ____________________
- Position of sternum: ____________________
- Sternal retraction: ____________________
- Slope of the ribs: ____________________
- Quality and pattern of respiration: ____________________
- Intercostal space: (retraction/bulging): ____________________
- Use of accessory muscle (sternomastoid/rectus abdominis): ____________________

Palpation:

- Sensation and tenderness (warm/cold sensation/pain/lesion/mass, etc.): ______
- Crepitus: ______
- Tactile fremitus (equal bilaterally): ______
- Assess the chest expansion: ______

Percussion:

- Tone (resonance/hyperresonance): ______
- Diaphragmatic excursion (normally 3–5 cm): ______

Auscultation:

- Breathing sound heard (normal/abnormal, crackles/wheezes/pleural friction/rub/stridor/any other, etc.):
  ______
- Breathing sound at: ______
- Vesicular: ______
- Bronchial: ______
- Bronchovesicular: ______
- Adventitious sound (present/absent): ______

CHEST INSPECTION

- Size and symmetry: ______
- Color and texture: ______
- Superficial venous pattern: ______
- Areola (color/size/shape/texture): ______
- Nipple (size/direction/discharge/lesion, etc.) ______
- Retraction or dimpling:

FEMALE BREAST

Palpation:

- Tenderness and temperature: ______
- Mass (size/location/shape, etc.): ______
- Nipple (discharge): ______
- Scar (mastectomy/lumpectomy): ______

AXILLA

Inspection and Palpation:

- Mass/tenderness/lesion, etc.: ______

MALE BREAST

Areolas, Nipple, and Axilla

Inspection and palpation:

- Any swelling include/nodule/discharge, etc.: ______

NECK

Inspection:

- Jugular venous pulses: ______

Auscultation and Palpation:

- Auscultate carotid artery (bruit/blowing/swishing sound): ______
- Palpate carotid artery (elasticity/thrillers): ______

HEART (PERICARDIUM)

Inspection:

- Pulsation (visible location): ______

Palpation:

- Apical impulses (present/absent/location): ______

Auscultation:

- Rate (per minute): Regular/irregular rhythm: ______
- S1 (lub) and S2 (dub) sound: ______
- Extra heart sound: ______

ARMS

Inspection:

- Color, size, venous pattern and edema: ______

Palpation:

- Fingers, hands, arms and warmth: ____________________
- Capillary refill time: ____________________
- Radial pulse (elasticity and strength): ____________________
- Ulnar pulse (present/absent): ____________________
- Brachial pulse (strength): ____________________
- Allen test: ____________________

LEGS

Inspection, Palpation and Auscultation:

- Distribution of hair: ____________________
- Any lesions or ulcer: ____________________
- Edema with characteristics: ____________________
- Varicosities temperature of feet and legs: ____________________
- On palpation of superficial inguinal lymph nodes: ____________________
- On palpation superficial pulse (amplifier and strength): ____________________
- On auscultation of femoral pulse (amplitude and strength): ____________________
- On palpation of popliteal pulse: ____________________
- On palpation of dorsalis pedis pulse (strong/weak/absent): ____________________
- On palpation posterior tibia pulses (strong/weak/absent: ____________________

ABDOMEN

Inspection

- Color of skin: ____________________
- Vascularity of the skin: ____________________
- Presence of scar: ____________________
- Assess for lesions and rashes: ____________________
- Observe for umbilical for skin color, location and contour: ____________________
- Abdominal contour (flat/rounded/scaphoid): ____________________
- Symmetry: ____________________
- Aortic pulsation: ____________________
- Peristaltic waves: ____________________
- Observable wave: ____________________

Auscultation:

Note: While doing the assessment of abdomen, auscultation is done before percussion and palpation, as their steps may alter the bowel sound.

- Bowel sound (intensity, pitch and frequency): ____________________
- Vascular sound (presence or absence of bruit sound): ____________________
- Venous rub over the spleen and liver: ____________________
- Friction rub over the spleen and liver: ____________________

Percussion:

- Percuss for tone (tympani and dull sound at different locations): ____________________
- The span or height of the liver: ____________________
- Spleen: ____________________
- Blunt percussion to find tenderness and muscular resistance: ____________________
- Deep palpation at all 4 quadrants to delineate abdominal organs and detect subtle masses: ____________________
- Assess for masses (in all quadrants): ____________________
- Umbilicus and surroundings: ____________________
- Liver (usually not palpable): ____________________
- Spleen (rarely palpable at left costal margin): ____________________
- Kidney (usually not palpable): ____________________
- Urinary bladder: ____________________

Special Test:

- Ascites (shifting dullness, fluid wave, etc.): ____________________
- Appendicitis (rebound tenderness, psoas sign, obturator sign, hypersensitivity test): ____________________

GAIT

Inspection:

- Patient's ability to walk and move around: ____________________
- Foot position, posture and arm swing during walk: ____________________
- Temporomandibular joint—inspection and palpation: ____________________
- Sternoclavicular joint—inspection and palpation: ____________________
- Cervical, thoracic and lumbar vertebra—inspection and palpation: ____________________

Movement of Cervical Spine:

- Flexion and hyperextension: __________
- Lateral bending: __________
- Rotation: __________

Movement of Thoracic and Lumbar Spine:

- Flexion and extension: __________
- Lateral bending: __________
- Rotation: __________
- Measure leg length: __________
- Straight leg test: __________

SHOULDER AND ARM

Inspection and Palpation:

- Assess for symmetry, color, swelling and masses: __________

Movement:

- Flexion and hyperextension: __________
- Adduction and abduction: __________
- External and internal rotation: __________

ELBOW

Inspection and Palpation:

- Assess size, shape, deformities, redness or swelling: __________

Movement:

- Flexion and extension: __________
- Supination and pronation: __________
- External and pronation: __________

WRIST

Inspection and Palpation:

- Assess size, shape symmetry, color, swelling: __________

- Presence of tenderness and nodules: ______
- Any tenderness in anatomical snuffbox: ______

Movement:

- Flexion and extension: ______
- Radial and ulnar deviation: ______
- Carpal tunnel syndrome: ______
- Phalen's test: ______
- Tinel's test: ______
- Flick test: ______
- Test for thumb weakness: ______

HANDS AND FINGERS

Inspection and Palpation:

- Assess size, shape symmetry, color, swelling: ______
- Palpate for tenderness, swelling bony prominence, nodules or crepitus: ______

Movement:

- Abduction and adduction: ______
- Flexion hyperextension: ______
- Internal and external hip rotation: ______

KNEE

Inspection and Palpation:

- Assess size, shape symmetry, swelling, deformities and alignment: ______
- On palpation knee (tenderness, warmth, consciousness, consistency nodule): ______

Movement:

- Flexion and hyperextension: ______
- Ballottement test: ______
- Mercury test: ______

ANKLES AND FEET

Inspection and Palpation:

- Assess patient in sitting, standing and walking for position, alignment, shape and skin of toe and feet: ____________
- Palpation of ankles and feet (tenderness, heat, swelling or nodule, pain): ____________
- Metatarsophalangeal joint (pain/tenderness): ____________

Movement:

- Dorsiflexion and plantarflexion of foot and ankle: ____________
- Eversion and inversion: ____________
- Abduction and adduction: ____________
- Flexion and extension: ____________

Reflexes:

	Biceps	Triceps	Brachioradialis	Patellar (quadriceps)	Achilles	Ankle clonus
Right side						
Left side						

Superficial Reflexes:

- Abdominal reflex: ____________
- Cremasteric reflex in male patient: ____________
- Test for meningeal irritation: ____________
- Brudziński's sign: ____________
- Kernig's sign: ____________

MALE GENITALIA

Penis

Inspection:

- Urinary catheter (present/absent): ____________________
- Inspect the base part of penis, pubic hairs, skin of the shaft, foreskin, glans: ____________________

Palpation:

- Palpate the shape for tenderness, pain, discharge, etc.____________________

Scrotum

Inspection:

- Inspect the shape, tenderness, and skin scrotum: ____________________

INGUINAL AREA

Inspection:

- Inspect the inguinal femoral areas for any bulge: ____________________

Palpation:

- Palpate on both side of inguinal area for lymph node, masses or bulging, femoral hernia: ____________________

____

FEMALE GENITALIA

External Genitalia

Inspection:

- Urinary catheter (present/absent): ____________________
- Assess the mons pubis, inguinal lymph, labia majora and perineum: ____________________
- Inspect the labia minora, clitoris, urethral meatus and vaginal opening: ____________________

Palpation:

- Bartholin gland (swelling, pain, discharge): ____________________
- Urethra (discharge, tenderness): ____________________

Internal Genitalia

Inspection:

- Observe the size and angle of vaginal opening: ____________________
- Assess vaginal musculature: ____________________
- Inspection of cervix (smoothness, color): ____________________
- Assess the vagina (redness, lesion, color, discharge): ____________________
- Bimanual examination (tenderness, lesion, pain): ____________________

Anus and Rectum

Inspection:

- Insect and opening area for lump, ulcer, lesion, rashes, redness, fissures, thickness of skin: ____________________
- Assess Valsalva maneuver: ____________________
- Assess sacrococcygeal area for swelling, redness, dimpling or hair, etc.: ____________________

Palpation:

- **Anus:** Any sphincter tightness, bleeding, pain, etc. ____________________
- **Rectum:** Presence of smoothness, tenderness, nodules, irregularities, etc.: ____________________
- **Prostate gland:** (normally nontender and rubbery): ____________________
- Inspect stool, if available: ____________________

INVESTIGATIONS

BLOOD/PATHOLOGICAL INVESTIGATIONS

Investigations	Normal values	Patient investigations values			Remark
		Date	Date	Date	
HEMATOLOGY					
Hemoglobin	12.5–17.5 g/dL				
RBC	4.50–6.0 × 10^6/mL				
PCV	35.0–50.4%				
MCV	80.0–99.9 fl				
MCH	27.0–31.0 pg.				
MCHC	33.0–37.0 g/dL				
Total WBC	4000–11000/cumm				
DLC: Polymorphs	40–75%				
Lymphocytes	20–40%				
Eosinophil	01–06%				
Monocytes	02–08%				
Basophil	00–01%				
Malaria parasite					
Smear: Normal					
Platelet count	1.5–4.5 lakhs/cumm				
ESR	Up to 15 mm at 1 hour				
AEC	40–440/cumm				
Retic count	0.5–2.5%				
Prothrombin time					
INR					
PTTK					
Bleeding time	1–5 minutes				
Clotting time	3–8 minutes				
Urine: Appearance					
Reaction					
Albumin					

Investigations	Normal values	Patient investigations values			Remark
		Date	Date	Date	
Sugar					
Acetone					
Bile salt/pigments					
Pus cells					
RBCs					
Others					
SEROLOGY: HIV					
HBsAg					
BIOCHEMISTRY					
Blood sugar fasting	70–110 mg/dL				
Postprandial	90–160 mg/dL				
Random	90–160 mg/dL				
HbA1c	4.2–6.2 mg/dL				
Blood urea	14–50 mg/dL				
Serum creatinine	0.6–1.4 mg/dL				
Uric acid	M: 2.7–7.7 mg/dL F: 2.4–5.7 mg/dL				
CPK	Up to 190 IU/L				
CPK MB	Up to 40 IU /L				
SGOT	Up to 40 IU/L				
LDH	Up to 450 IU /L				
Serum sodium	134–148 mEq /L				
Serum potassium	3.5–5.6 mEq/L				
Serum calcium	8.1–10.4 mg/dL				
Serum phosphorous	2.5–4.5 mg/dL				
Serum magnesium	1.8–2.6 mg/dL				
LIPID: Total cholesterol	Up to 200 mg/dL				
HDL cholesterol	40–60 mg/dL				
Serum triglycerides	Up to 150 mg/dL				
LDL cholesterol	Up to 100 mg/dL				

Investigations	Normal values	Patient investigations values			Remark
		Date	Date	Date	
LFT: Total protein	6.0–7.8 g/dL				
Albumin	3.2–4.5 g/dL				
Globulin	2.3–3.5 g/dL				
Bilirubin total	Up to 1.2 mg/dL				
Bilirubin direct	Up to 0.25 mg/dL				
SGPT	Up to 40 IU/L				
Alkaline phosphates	Up to 150 IU/L				
Serum digoxin	0.8–2.0 ng/mL				
Serum amylase	25–125 U/L				
SEROLOGY					
RA:					
CRP:					
ASO:					
TROP- T					

OTHER DIAGNOSTIC INVESTIGATIONS:

Ultrasonography (USG): (abdomen/pelvis/kidney/urethra/bladder (kub) etc.):

____

X-ray: (abdomen/pelvis/kidney/urethra/bladder (KUB) etc.):

____

Computer tomography (CT scan):

____

Magnetic resonance imagination: (MRI):

____

Any other:

____

MEDICATION

Sl. no.	Name of medication, route, dose	Action	Indication	Contraindication	Side effects	Nurses responsibility

LIST OF NURSING DIAGNOSIS ACCORDING TO PRIORITY

NURSING CARE PLAN

Assessment	Nursing diagnosis	Expected outcome	Planning intervention	Rationale	Evaluation
Subjective data: **Objective data:**		**Short-term outcome:** **Long-term outcome:**			

NURSING CARE PLAN

Assessment	Nursing diagnosis	Expected outcome	Planning intervention	Rationale	Evaluation
Subjective data:		**Short-term outcome:**			
Objective data:		**Long-term outcome:**			

NURSING CARE PLAN

Assessment	Nursing diagnosis	Expected outcome	Planning intervention	Rationale	Evaluation
Subjective data:		**Short-term outcome:**			
Objective data:		**Long-term outcome:**			

NURSING CARE PLAN

Assessment	Nursing diagnosis	Expected outcome	Planning intervention	Rationale	Evaluation
Subjective data:		**Short-term outcome:**			
Objective data:		**Long-term outcome:**			

HEALTH EDUCATION

Disease condition: ______________________________

Diet: ______________________________

Personal hygiene: ______________________________

Medication: ______________________________

Lifestyle modification: ______________________________

Follow-up care: ______________________________

BIBLIOGRAPHY/REFERENCES

(Write bibliography in the Vancouver style)

EVALUATION PROFORMA NURSING PROCESS

Name of the Student: ______________________ **Date:** ____________

Clinical Area: ______________________ **Diagnosis:** ____________

Sl. no.	Criteria	Allotted marks	Obtained marks
1	History collection	3	
2	Physical examination	3	
3	Drug study	2	
4	Nursing assessment	2	
5	Prioritize the nursing diagnosis	5	
6	Nursing care plan on 5 need-based nursing diagnosis	5	
7	Prognosis of patient	1	
8	Nurses notes	2	
9	Bibliography/References	2	
Total		**25**	

Remarks: ______________________

Signature of the Student **Signature of the Evaluator**

PRESSURE SORE ASSESSMENT

Name of the Patient: ____________________ **Gender:** ____________________

Ward/Unit: ____________________ **Admission Date:** ____________________

Diagnosis: ____________________

Criteria	1	2	3	4	Patients score
Sensory perception: Ability to respond meaningfully to pressure related discomfort.	**Completed limited:** Unresponsiveness to painful stimuli due to diminished level of consciousness or solution or limited ability to feel pain over most body surface.	**Very limited:** Responds only to painful stimuli or has impairment which limits the ability to feel pain or discomfort over ½ of the body.	**Slightly limited:** Responds to verbal commands but cannot always communicably discomfort or need to be turned OR has some sensory impairment which limits ability to feel pain or discomfort in 1 or 2 extremities.	**No impairment:** Responds to verbal commands. Has no sensory deficit to feel or voice pain to discomfort.	
Moisture: Degree to which skin is exposed to moisture.	**Constantly moist:** Skin is moist constantly by respiration, urine, etc. dampness is detected every time patient is moved or turned.	**Very moist:** Skin is often but not constantly moist. Linen must be changed at least once a shift.	**Occasionally moist:** Skin is occasionally moist, requires changing approximately once a day.	**Rarely moist:** Skin is usually dry. Linen only requires changing at routine intervals.	
Activity: Degree of physical activity.	**Bedfast:** Confirmed to bed.	**Chair fast:** Ability to walk severely limited or non-existent cannot bear own weight or must be assisted into chair wheelchair.	**Walk occasionally:** For short distance with or without assistance spends majority of time without assistance.	**Walk frequently:** Walks outside the room at least twice a day and inside room at least once every 2 hours during walking hours.	
Mobility: Ability to change and control body position.	**Completely immobile:** Does not make even slight changes in body extremity position without assistance.	**Very limited:** Occasional slight changes in body or extremity position but unable to make frequent or significant changes independently.	**Slight limited:** Makes frequent slight changes in body or extremity position independently.	**No limitation:** Makes major and frequent changes in position without assistance.	

Contd...

Criteria	1	2	3	4	Patients score
Nutrition: Usual food intake pattern.	**Very poor:** Never eats a complete meal. Rarely eats more than 1/3rd of any food offered. Eats 2 servings or less of proteins per day. Fluids taken poorly does not take a liquid dietary supplement or in NBM and/or maintained on clear liquid or IVs for more than 5 days.	**Probably inadequate:** Rarely eats complete meals and generally eats only ½ of any food offered. Protein intake includes only 3 servings of meat or dairy products per day. Occasionally will take a dairy supplement OR received less than optimum of liquid diet or tube feeding.	**Adequate:** Eats over half meals, eats a total of 4 servings or protein each day. Occasionally will refuse a meal, but will usually take a supplement if offered or is on a tube feeding or TPN regimen which probably meets most of nutrition needs.	**Excellent:** Eats most in every meal. Never refuses a meal. Usually eats a total 4 or more servings of meal and dairy products. Occasionally eats between meals. Does not require supplementations.	
Friction and shear	**Problem:** Requires moderate to maximum assistance in moving. Complete lifting without sliding against sheets is impossible. Frequently slides sheets in bed or chair, requiring frequent repositioning with maximum assistance or agitation leads to almost constant friction.	**Potential problems:** Moves feebly or requires minimum assistance. During a move skin probably slides to some extent against sheets. Chair restraints or other devices maintain good position in bed or chair, but occasionally slides down.	**No apparent problems:** Moves in bed and chair independently, has sufficient muscle strength to lift up completely during move. Maintains good position in bed or chair at all times.	–	
Total score					**23**

Note: Patient with total score of 18 or less are considered to be risk of developing pressure ulcer.
(19–23 No risk, 15–18 Low risk, 13–14 = Moderate risk, 10–12 = High risk, <9 = Very high risk)
(This Braden pressure ulcer risk assessment card is for Basic BSc Nursing students practicing nursing in the clinical area.)

Overall findings:

Signature of the Student

Signature of the Supervisor

EVALUATION PROFORMA PRESSURE SORE ASSESSMENT

Name of the Student: ______________________

Ward/Unit: ______________________

Date of Submission/Presentation: ______________________

Sl. no	Evaluation criteria	Maximum marks	Marks obtained
1.	Identification of patient	05	
2.	Assessment of pressure sore	05	
3.	Applies care modalities while prevention pressure sore	05	
4.	Rapport with the patients	05	
5.	Recording and reporting	05	
Total		**25**	

Remarks: ______________________

Signature of the Student

Signature of the Supervisor/Evaluator

FALL RISK ASSESSMENT

Name of the Patient: ______________________ **Gender:** __________

Ward/Unit: ______________________ **Admission Date:** __________

Diagnosis: ______________________

Risk factors	**Rating scale**				
	0	**1**	**2**	**3**	**Rating score**
Age	16–65 years	65–70 years	70–79 years	>80 years	
Falls history	No fall in last year.	1 or more falls over last 3–6 months.	2 or more falls within last 3 months.	3 or more falls while inpatient.	
Mobility/activity and balance	Ambulates without assistance.	Ambulates without assistance but with a gait aid and steady gait.	Ambulates with or without assistance –occasionally unsteady.	Ambulates with or without assistance—unsteady at all times immobile/ bed rest.	
Mental state	Oriented to time, place, and person.	Oriented to place and person only.	Oriented to person only.	Disoriented and/or impaired judgment and/or impulsive.	
Sensory	Normal	Requires glasses or hearing aid.	Recent surgery or sensory deficit with or without aid in use.	Legally blind or deaf.	
Medication: • Antihypertensive • Vasodilators • Diuretics • Antiparkinsonians • Vestibular depressants	NIL	Takes 1–2 listed medications.	Takes 3 or more listed medications.	Postural hypotension related to medication.	
Continence	Continent	Increased frequency	Nocturnal or stress incontinence/ indwelling catheters.	Urge incontinence.	

(If the total score is 2 or more, or if the patient falls at any time of their admission, please complete the falls prevention checklist and action plan.)

Date:

______________________ ______________

Name of the Student **Signature**

FALLS RISK ASSESSMENT TOOL PREVENTION STRATEGIES

Environment	Mental state	Mobility/sensory
• Bed in lowest position • Obstacles/excess furniture removed • Personal items/call bell within reach • Wheel brakes applied as needed • Room near nurses' station • Rest points (chairs) provided • Night lights provided • Use of appropriate equipment (e.g., shower chair) • Use Hi-Lo bed • Appropriate height of chairs	• Regular reorientation provided • Information given clearly and slowly • Reassurance provided regularly • Noise reduced in immediate area • "Traffic" reduced in immediate area • Specialist referral (psych) as needed	• Use of appropriate footwear • Sensory aids worn as needed • Alert label applied to mobility aid • Provide appropriate level of assistance (specify)
Continence	**Medications**	**Other measures**
• Regular toileting times established • Fluid balance recorded • Continence records utilized (if available) • Timing of laxatives and diuretics checked • Commode chair provided • Referred to continence services	• Full review completed on admission • Medication reviews repeated post fall • Dosages and combinations checked • Postural hypotension reviewed	• Review hydration/nutrition • Apply hip protectors Referral to: • Physiotherapist • Occupational therapist • Dietitian

FALLS PREVENTION CHECKLIST AND ACTION PLAN

Name of the Patient: ____________________ **Hospital Number:** __________

Name of Student Nurse: ____________________ **Ward:** __________

Date and time	Risk factors	Action to be taken	Reassessment	Action to be taken if factors have changed
	The patient needs to use the toilet more than four hourly.	If yes, ensure that they are positioned close enough to the toilet which is a distance of........		
	Footwear is well fitting and suitable.	Ensure footwear is worn when the patient is out of bed. If footwear is unsuitable, arrange replacement.		
	Lying and standing blood pressure has systolic drop of 20 mm Hg and/or reports dizziness on standing	If yes, discuss with medical staff and take action.		
	Prescribed medication is predictive of falls, sedatives, antidepressants, antipsychotics.	If yes, discuss with medical staff.		
	Patient has significant cognitive impairment, e.g., appears unaware of risk of falling.	If yes, position close to the nurse's station.		
	Patient appears agitated.	If yes, provide close supervision, avoid centrally acting medication, and ensure adequate lighting.		
	Other contributory factors are present: Constipation, infection, drug withdrawal, (alcohol, benzodiazepines) dementia.	If yes, state which factors and action to be taken.		
	Environmental factors to be checked at each patient intervention.	Ensure that the call bell is working, within reach and that the patient knows how to use it. Ensure that the bed is at the lowest height and that the brakes are on. Ensure that the bed area is free from hazards, e.g., clutter, wet floors, trailing wires. Ensure that the patients' belongings and any aids and equipment are within reach. Ensure that the chair is at the correct height for the patient which is .... cm. Ensure that night-lights are used at night.		

For patients who are identified as at risk of falls.

EVALUATION PROFORMA FALL RISK ASSESSMENT

Name of the Student: ______________________

Ward/Unit: ______________________

Date of Submission/Presentation: ______________________

Sl. no	Evaluation criteria	Maximum marks	Marks obtained
1.	Identification of patient	05	
2.	Assessment of fall risk	05	
3.	Applies care modalities for prevention of fall risk	05	
4.	Rapport with the patients	05	
5.	Recording and reporting	05	
Total		**25**	

Remarks: ______________________

Signature of the Student

Signature of Supervisor/Evaluator

CLINICAL EXPERIENCE DETAILS

Name of the clinical areas	Clinical condition	Number of days care given	Signature of Faculty/Preceptor

Signature of the Faculty Coordinator

Signature of the HOD/Principal

Signature of the Internal Examiner

Name: ____________________

Date: ____________________

Signature of the External Examiner

Name: ____________________

Date: ____________________

Supplementary Examination:

Signature of the Internal Examiner

Name: ____________________

Date: ____________________

Signature of the External Examiner

Name: ____________________

Date: ____________________

ANNEXURES

ABBREVIATIONS

- **ABG** Arterial blood gas
- **ABCDE** Airway, breathing, circulation, disability, expose and examine
- **A.C.** Before meal (ante cibum)
- **AIDS** Acquired immunodeficiency syndrome
- **AD** As desired
- **ADL** Activities of daily living
- **AI** Adequate intake
- **BUN** Blood urea nitrogen
- **CBC** Complete blood count
- **CC** Cubic centimeter
- **CO_2** Carbon dioxide
- **CSF** Cerebrospinal fluid
- **Dx** Diagnosis
- **ENT** Eye, ear, nose, throat
- **ECG** Electrocardiogram
- **G or Gm** Gram
- **gt.** Drop (gutte)
- **HCl** Hydrochloric acid
- **HS** At bed-time (hours of sleep)
- **NPO** Nothing by mouth
- **IVP** Intravenous pyelogram
- **KI** Potassium iodide
- **NaCl** Sodium chloride
- **QH** Every hour
- **QD** Every day
- **RBC** Red blood count or red blood cell
- **Rh** Rhesus factor
- **BP** Blood pressure
- **BMR** Basal metabolic rate
- **BM** Bowel movement
- **BID** Twice a day (bis in die)
- **Ax** Axillary
- **AMA** Against medical advice
- **AMALG** Amalgam filling
- **CXR** Chest X-ray
- **D and C** Dilatation and curettage
- **DPT** Diphtheria, pertussis, tetanus
- **D/W** Dextrose in water
- **EEG** Electroencephalogram
- **°F** Fahrenheit
- **FBS** Fasting blood sugar
- **FHB** Fetal heartbeat
- **GI** Gastrointestinal
- **gtt.** Drops
- **Hb** Hemoglobin
- **IV** Intravenous
- **Rx** Prescription, take
- **LP** Lumbar puncture
- **OPD** Out patient department
- **OR** Operating room
- **PRN** As needed, when necessary
- **QID** Four times a day
- **QOD** Every other day
- **SOS** If necessary

- **STAT** Immediately at once
- **TPR** Temperature, pulse, respiration
- **Tsp** Teaspoon, tablespoon
- **Wt** Weight
- **URQ** Upper right quadrant
- **NG** Nasogastric
- **PTT** Partial thromboplastin time
- **RNA** Ribonucleic acid
- **ECG** Electrocardiogram
- **HIV** Human immunodeficiency virus
- **HPV** Human papilloma virus
- **HSV** Herpes simplex virus
- **IgA** Immunoglobulin A
- **IgE** Immunoglobulin E
- **MI** Myocardial infarction
- **AST** Aspartate aminotransferase
- **SC** Subcutaneous
- **TID** Three times a day
- **WBC** White blood cells
- **ULQ** Upper lower quadrant
- **UTI** Urinary tract infection
- **OTC** Over the counter
- **PTCA** Percutaneous transluminal coronary angioplasty
- **REM** Rapid eye movement
- **stat** Immediately
- **EEG** Electroencephalogram
- **GABA** Gamma aminobutyric acid
- **GFR** Glomerular filtration rate
- **ICP** Intracranial pressure
- **LD** Lactate dehydrogenase
- **LOC** Lactated ringer's solution
- **ACE** Angiotensin-converting enzyme

TERMINOLOGY

- **Abduction:** Movement away from the center or median line of the body.
- **Acute pain:** Pain that is generally rapid in onset and varies in intensity from mild to severe.
- **Adduction:** Movement toward the center or median line of the body.
- **Adjuvant:** Substances or treatments that enhance the effect of another treatment; especially substances that enhance the effect of drugs.
- **Adventitious breath sounds:** Sounds that are not normally heard in the lungs on auscultation.
- **Adverse drug effect:** Undesirable effects other than the intended therapeutic effect in medication administration.
- **Alopecia:** Baldness.
- **Alveoli:** Small air sacs at the end of the terminal bronchioles that are the site of gas exchange.
- **Ampule:** A glass flask that contains a single dose of medication for parenteral administration.
- **Analgesic:** Agent used to relieve pain.
- **Anesthetic:** Medication that produces such states as narcosis (loss of consciousness), analgesia, relaxation, and loss of reflexes.
- **Approximated wound edges:** Edges of a wound that are lightly pulled together; epithelialization of wound margins; edges touch, wound is closed.
- **Arterial blood gas (ABG):** A laboratory test that evaluates the oxygen, carbon dioxide, bicarbonate, and pH of an arterial blood sample, determining metabolic or respiratory alkalosis or acidosis.
- **Arteriovenous fistula:** A surgically created passage connecting an artery and a vein, used in hemodialysis.
- **Arteriovenous graft:** A surgically created connection between an artery and vein using synthetic material; used in hemodialysis.
- **Arthroplasty:** Surgical formation or reformation of a joint.
- **Aspiration:** The misdirection of oropharyngeal secretions or gastric contents into the larynx and lower respiratory tract.
- **Atelectasis:** *Inc*omplete expansion or collapse of a part of the lungs.
- **Atelectasis:** Incomplete expansion or collapse of a part of the lungs.
- **Aura:** A premonitory or warning sensation of a seizure that can be visual, auditory, or olfactory.
- **Auscultation:** Act of listening with a stethoscope to sounds produced within the body.
- **Autologous transfusion:** A blood transfusion donated by the patient in anticipation that he or she may need the transfusion during a hospital stay.
- **Body mass index (BMI):** Ratio of height to weight that more accurately reflects total body fat stores in the general population (weight in kg/height in meters).
- **Breakthrough pain:** A temporary flare-up of moderate to severe pain that occurs even when the patient is taking around-the-clock medication for persistent pain.
- **Bruit:** A sound caused by turbulent blood flow.
- **Bruits:** Abnormal "swooshing" sounds heard on auscultation, indicating turbulent blood flow.
- **Calorie:** Measure of heatw, or energy; kilocalorie, commonly referred to as a calorie, is defined as the amount of heat required to raise 1 kg of water by 1C.
- **Carbohydrate:** Organic compounds (commonly known as sugars and starches) that are composed of carbon, hydrogen, and oxygen; the most abundant and least expensive source of calories in the diet worldwide.
- **Cardiac arrest:** Sudden cessation of functional circulation of the heart (pulse), such as asystole or defibrillation, typically caused by the occlusion of one or more of the coronary arteries or cardiomyopathies.
- **Cardiac monitoring:** Visualization and monitoring of the cardiac electrical activity stimulating the heartbeat.
- **Cardiopulmonary resuscitation (CPR):** Also known as basic life support; revival in the absence of spontaneous respirations and heartbeat to preserve heart and brain function while waiting for defibrillation and advanced cardiac life support care. Achieved by manually pumping the heart by compressing the sternum and forcing oxygen into the lungs using mouth-to-mouth or rescue breathing.

- **Cardioversion:** Conversion of a pathologic cardiac rhythm to normal sinus rhythm through low doses of electricity, using a device that applies synchronized countershocks to the heart.
- **Caries:** Cavities of the teeth.
- **Central venous access device (CVAD):** A venous access device in which the tip of the catheter terminates in the central venous circulation, usually in the superior vena cava just above the right atrium.
- **Cerebral perfusion pressure (CPP):** A way of calculating cerebral blood flow; the formula is MAP (mean arterial pressure) minus ICP (intracranial pressure) equals CPP; normal CPP for an adult is 60–90 mm Hg.
- **Cerumen:** Ear wax; consists of a heavy oil and brown pigmentation.
- **Cholesterol:** Fatlike substance, found only in animal tissues, that is important for cell membrane structure, a precursor of steroid hormones, and a constituent of bile.
- **Chronic pain:** Pain that may be limited, intermittent, or persistent but lasts beyond the normal healing period.
- **Cilia:** Microscopic, hair-like projections that propel mucus toward the upper airway so that it can be expectorated.
- **Colostomy:** Artificial opening that permits feces from the colon to exit through the stoma.
- **Coma:** A pathologic state of unconsciousness characterized by an unarousable sleep like state; eyes closed at all times; no speech or sound noted; no spontaneous movement of extremities.
- **Compartment syndrome:** Occurs when there is increased tissue pressure within a limited space; leads to compromises in the circulation and the function of the involved tissue.
- **Consciousness:** The degree of wakefulness or ability to be aroused.
- **Conscious sedation/analgesia:** Type of anesthesia used for short procedures; the intravenous administration of sedatives and analgesics raises the pain threshold and produces an altered mood and some degree of amnesia, but the patient maintains cardiopulmonary function and can respond to verbal commands.
- **Constipation:** Passage of dry, hard stools.
- **Continuous wound perfusion pain management system:** Device that delivers a continuous infusion of local analgesia to a surgical wound bed.
- **Contracture:** Permanent shortening or tightening of a muscle due to spasm or paralysis.
- **Contusion:** An injury in which the skin is not broken; a bruise.
- **Crossmatching:** Determining the compatibility of two blood specimens.
- **Cyanosis:** Bluish or greyish discoloration of the skin in response to inadequate oxygenation.
- **Debridement:** Removal of devitalized tissue and foreign material from a wound.
- **Deep-vein thrombosis:** A blood clot in a blood vessel originating in the large veins of the legs.
- **Defecation:** Emptying of the large intestine; also called a bowel movement.
- **Defibrillation:** Stopping fibrillation of the heart by using an electrical device that applies countershocks to the heart through electrodes on the chest wall. This countershock is given in an attempt to allow the heart's normal pacemaker to take over.
- **Dehiscence:** Accidental separation of wound edges, especially a surgical wound.
- **Dehydration:** Decreased fluid volume.
- **Diarrhea:** Passage of excessively liquid, unformed stool.
- **Dysphagia:** Difficulty swallowing or the inability to swallow.
- **Dyspnea:** Difficult or labored breathing.
- **Ecchymosis:** A collection of blood in the subcutaneous tissues, causing purplish discoloration.
- **Ecchymosis:** Discoloration of an area resulting from infiltration of blood into the subcutaneous tissue.
- **Edema:** Accumulation of fluid in body tissues.
- **Edema:** Accumulation of fluid in the interstitial tissues.
- **Edema:** Excess fluid in the tissues, characterized by swelling.
- **Elective surgery:** Surgery that is recommended but can be omitted or delayed without a negative effect.
- **Electrocardiogram (ECG/EKG):** Graphing of the electrical activity of the heart.
- **Embolus:** Foreign body or air in the circulatory system.
- **Endotracheal tube:** Polyvinylchloride airway that is inserted through the nose or mouth into the trachea, using a laryngoscope.

- **Enema:** Introduction of a solution into the large intestine.
- **Enteral nutrition:** Alternate form of feeding that involves passing a tube into the gastrointestinal tract to allow instillation of the appropriate formula.
- **Epidural route:** Administration of analgesia via an infusion catheter placed in the epidural space.
- **Epithelialization:** Stage of wound healing in which epithelial cells move across the surface of a wound margin (approximation); tissue color ranges from the color of "ground glass" to pink.
- **Erythema:** Redness of the skin.
- **Erythema:** Redness or inflammation of an area as a result of dilation and congestion of capillaries.
- **Eschar:** A thick, leathery scab or dry crust composed of dead cells and dried plasma.
- **Expiration:** Act of breathing out.
- **Extension:** The return movement from flexion; the joint angle is increased.
- **External condom catheter:** Soft, pliable sheath made of silicone material, applied externally to the penis, connected to drainage tubing and a collection bag.
- **Extubation:** Removal of a tube (in this case, an endotracheal tube).
- **Exudate:** Fluid that accumulates in a wound; may contain serum, cellular debris, bacteria, and white blood cells.
- **Fecal impaction:** Prolonged retention or an accumulation of fecal material that forms a hardened mass in the rectum.
- **Fenestrated:** Having a window-like opening.
- **Fibrillation:** Small, local, involuntary contraction of muscle, resulting from spontaneous activation of a single muscle fiber or of an isolated bundle of nerve fibers.
- **Flatus:** Intestinal gas.
- **Flexion:** Bending of a joint so that the angle of the joint diminishes.
- **Fracture:** A break in the continuity of the bone.
- **General survey:** Overall impression of a person by the health care provider; includes physical appearance, body structure, mobility, and behavior.
- **Gingivitis:** Inflammation of the gingivae (gums).
- **Goniometer:** An apparatus to measure joint movement and angles.
- **Granulation tissue:** New tissue that is deep pink/red and composed of fibroblasts and small blood vessels that fill an open wound when it starts to heal; characterized by irregular surface like raspberries.
- **Halitosis:** Offensive breath.
- **Healthcare-associated infection:** Infection not present on admission to healthcare agency; acquired during the course of treatment for other conditions.
- **Hemodialysis:** Removal from the body, by means of blood filtration, of toxins and fluid that are normally removed by the kidneys.
- **Hemorrhage:** Excessive blood loss due to the escape of blood from blood vessels.
- **Hemorrhoids:** Abnormally distended veins in the anal area.
- **Hemothorax:** Blood in the pleural space around the heart.
- **Hyperextension:** Extreme or abnormal extension.
- **Hypertonic:** Having a greater concentration of solutes than the solution with which it is being compared.
- **Hyperventilation:** Condition in which more than the normal amount of air is entering and leaving the lungs as a result of an increase in rate or depth of respiration or both.
- **Hypervolemia:** Excess of isotonic fluid (water and sodium) in the extracellular space.
- **Hypothermia:** Condition characterized by a body temperature below 96.8F.
- **Hypotonic:** Having a lesser concentration than the solution with which it is being compared.
- **Hypoventilation:** Decreased rate or depth of air movement into the lungs.
- **Hypovolemia:** Deficiency of isotonic fluid (water and sodium) from the extracellular space.
- **Hypovolemic shock:** Shock due to a decrease in blood volume.
- **Hypoxia:** Inadequate amount of oxygen available to the cells.

- **Ileal conduit:** A surgical diversion formed by bringing the ureters to the ileum; urine is excreted through a stoma.
- **Ileostomy:** Artificial opening created to allow liquid fecal content from the ileum to be eliminated through a stoma.
- **Implanted port:** A type of CVAD; subcutaneous injection port attached to a catheter; distal catheter tip dwells in the lower one third of the superior vena cava to the junction of the superior vena cava and the right atrium and the proximal end or port is usually implanted in a subcutaneous pocket of the upper chest wall. Implanted ports placed in the antecubital area of the arm are referred to as peripheral access system ports.
- **Indwelling urethral catheter (retention or Foley catheter):** A catheter (tube) through the urethra into the bladder for the purpose of continuous drainage of urine; a balloon is inflated to ensure that the catheter remains in the bladder once it is inserted.
- **Inhalation:** Route to administer medications directly into the lungs or airway passages.
- **Inspection:** Process of performing deliberate, purposeful observations in a systematic manner.
- **Inspiration:** Act of breathing in.
- **Integument:** Skin.
- **Intermittent urethral catheter (straight catheter):** A catheter through the urethra into the bladder to drain urine for a short period of time (5–10 minutes).
- **Intracranial pressure (ICP):** Pressure within the cranial vault; normal ICP is less than 10–15 mm Hg.
- **Intractable pain:** Pain that is resistant to therapy and persists despite a variety of interventions.
- **Intradermal injection:** Injection placed just below the epidermis; sites commonly used are the inner surface of the forearm, the dorsal aspect of the upper arm, and the upper back.
- **Intramuscular injection:** Injection placed into muscular tissue; sites commonly used are the ventrogluteal, vastus lateralis, deltoid, and dorsogluteal muscles.
- **Intravenous (IV) route:** Route to administer medication directly into the vein or venous system; the most dangerous route of medication administration.
- **Ischemia:** Insufficient blood supply to a body part due to obstruction of circulation.
- **Isotonic:** Having about the same solute concentration as the solution with which it is being compared.
- **Jaundice:** Condition characterized by yellowness of the skin, whites of eyes, mucous membranes, and body fluids as a result of deposition of bile pigment resulting from excess bilirubin in the blood.
- **Ketosis:** Catabolism of fatty acids that occurs when an individual's carbohydrate intake is not adequate; without adequate glucose, the catabolism is incomplete and ketones are formed, resulting in increased ketones.
- **Lipid:** Group name for fatty substances, including fats, oils, waxes, and related compounds.
- **Maceration:** Softening of tissue due to excessive moisture.
- **Medical asepsis:** Clean technique; involves procedures and practices that reduce the number and transfer of pathogens.
- **Metered-dose inhaler (MDI):** Device to deliver a controlled dose of medication for inhalation.
- **Minerals:** Inorganic elements found in nature.
- **Nasal cannula:** Disposable plastic device with two protruding prongs for insertion into the nostrils; used to administer oxygen.
- **Nasogastric (NG) tube:** A tube inserted through the nose and into the stomach.
- **Nasopharyngeal airway (nasal trumpet):** A curved, soft rubber or plastic tube inserted into the back of the pharynx through the mouth.
- **Nebulizer:** Instrument that produces a fine spray or mist; in this case, passing air through a liquid medication to produce fine particles for inhalation.
- **Necrosis:** Localized tissue death.
- **Needle gauge:** Measurement of the diameter of a needle.
- **Neuropathic pain:** Pain that results from an injury to or abnormal functioning of peripheral nerves or the central nervous system.
- **Nonintentional (NI) tube:** A tube inserted through the nose and into the upper portion of the small intestine.
- **Nonpharmacologic interventions:** Interventions without the use of medicine or drugs; interventions in addition to the use of medicines or drugs.

- **Nonsterile (clean) techniques:** Strategies used in patient care to reduce overall number of microorganisms or to prevent or reduce the risk of transmission of microorganisms from one person to another or from one place to another. Involve meticulous handwashing, maintaining a clean environment by preparing a clean field, using clean gloves and sterile instruments, and preventing direct contamination of materials and supplies.
- **Nosocomial infection:** Infection acquired while receiving health care.
- **NPO (nothing by mouth):** Nothing can be consumed by mouth, including medications, unless ordered otherwise.
- **Nutrient:** Specific biochemical substance used by the body for growth, development, activity, reproduction, lactation, health maintenance, and recovery from illness or injury.
- **Nutrition:** Study of the nutrients and how they are handled by the body, as well as the impact of human behavior and environment on the process of nourishment.
- **Obesity:** Weight greater than 20% above ideal body weight.
- **Oropharyngeal airway:** A semi-circular tube of plastic or rubber inserted into the back of the pharynx through the mouth.
- **Orthostatic hypotension:** An abnormal drop in blood pressure that occurs as a person changes from a supine to a standing position.
- **Ostomy:** A surgically formed opening from the inside of an organ to the outside.
- **Pain threshold:** The lowest intensity of a stimulus that causes the subject to recognize pain.
- **Pain tolerance:** Point beyond which a person is no longer willing to endure pain.
- **Pathogens:** Microorganisms that can harm humans.
- **Patient care ergonomics:** The practice of designing equipment and work tasks to conform to the capability of the worker in relation to patient care. It provides a means for adjusting the work environment and work practices to prevent injuries before they occur and is part of best practices for providing safe patient care.
- **Pediculosis:** Infestation with lice.
- **Percutaneous endoscopic gastrostomy tube (PEG):** A surgically or laparoscopically placed gastrostomy tube.
- **Percutaneous endoscopic jejunostomy tube (PEJ):** A surgically or laparoscopically placed jejunostomy tube.
- **Perfusion:** The process by which oxygenated capillary blood passes through the tissues of the body.
- **Perineural route:** Administration of local anesthetic for pain management via an infusion catheter placed along.
- **Perioperative nursing:** Wide variety of nursing activities carried out before, during, and after surgery.
- **Peripheral vascular disease:** Pathologic conditions of the vascular system characterized by reduced blood flow through the peripheral blood vessels.
- **Peripheral venous access device:** A short (less than 3 inches) peripheral catheter placed in a peripheral vein for short-term therapy. This device is not appropriate for certain therapies, such as vesicant chemotherapy, drugs that are classified as irritants, or TPN.
- **Peritoneal dialysis:** Removal of toxins and fluid from the body by the principles of diffusion and osmosis; accomplished by introducing a solution (dialysate) into the peritoneal cavity.
- **Peritonitis:** Inflammation of the peritoneal membrane.
- **Personal protective equipment (PPE):** Equipment and supplies necessary to minimize or prevent exposure to infectious material, including gloves, gowns, masks, and protective eye gear.
- **Plaque:** Transparent, adhesive coating on teeth consisting of mucin, carbohydrate, and bacteria.
- **Pleurae:** Membranes that cover the lungs.
- **Pleural effusion:** Fluid in the pleural space.
- **Pneumothorax:** Air in the pleural space.
- **Pressure ulcer:** Lesion caused by unrelieved pressure that results in damage to underlying tissue.
- **Pronation:** The act of lying face downward; the act of turning the hand so the palm faces downward or backward.
- **Protein:** Vital component of every living cell; composed of carbon, hydrogen, oxygen, and nitrogen.
- **Pulse oximetry:** Non-invasive technique that measures the oxygen saturation (SpO_2) of arterial blood.
- **Pyorrhea:** Extensive inflammation of the gums and alveolar tissues; synonym for periodontitis.
- **Recommended dietary allowance (RDA):** Recommendations for average daily amounts of essential nutrients that healthy people should consume over time.

- **Residual:** As applied to tube feeding, the amount of gastric contents in the stomach after the administration of a tube feeding.
- **Respiration:** Gas exchange between the atmospheric air in the alveoli and the blood in the capillaries.
- **Rotation:** Process of turning on an axis; twisting or revolving.
- **Sediment:** Precipitate found at the bottom of a container of urine.
- **Seizure:** Temporary alteration in brain function due to excessive and abnorma, electrical discharges of neurons in the brain that may result in uncontrolled body movements or a convulsion and alteration of consciousness.
- **Shearing force:** Force created by the interplay of gravity and friction on the skin and underlying tissues; shear causes tissue layers to slide over one another and blood vessels to stretch and twist and disrupts the microcirculation of the skin and subcutaneous tissue.
- **Sinus tract:** Cavity or channel underneath a wound that has the potential for infection.
- **Spirometer:** Instrument used to measure lung capacity and volume; one type is used to encourage deep breathing (incentive spirometry).
- **Standard precautions:** Precautions used in the care of all hospitalized individuals regardless of their diagnosis or possible infection status; these precautions apply to blood, all body fluids, secretions and excretions (except sweat), non-intact skin, and mucous membranes.
- **Sterile techniques:** Strategies used in patient care to reduce exposure to microorganisms and maintain objects and areas as free from microorganisms as possible. Involve meticulous handwashing, use of a sterile field, use of sterile gloves for application of a sterile dressing, and use of sterile instruments.
- **Stoma:** Artificial opening on the body surface.
- **Stoma:** The part of the ostomy that is attached to the skin; formed by suturing the mucosa to the skin.
- **Subcutaneous emphysema:** Small pockets of air trapped in the subcutaneous tissue; usually found around chest tube insertion sites.
- **Subcutaneous injection:** Injection placed between the epidermis and muscle, into the subcutaneous tissue; sites commonly used are the outer aspect of the upper arm, the abdomen, the anterior aspects of the thigh, the upper back, and the upper ventral or dorsogluteal area.
- **Supination:** Turning of the palm or foot upward.
- **Suppository:** Oval or cone-shaped substance that is inserted into a body cavity and melts at body temperature.
- **Suprapubic urinary catheter:** A urinary catheter surgically inserted through a small incision above the pubic area into the bladder.
- **Surgical asepsis:** Sterile technique; involves practices used to render and keep objects and areas free from microorganisms
- **Surgical staples:** Stainless-steel wire (shaped like a staple) used to close a surgical wound.
- **Surgical sutures:** Thread or wire used to hold tissue and skin together.
- **Symphysis pubis:** The anterior midline junction of the pubic bones; the bony projection under the pubic hair.
- **Tachypnea:** Rapid breathing.
- **Tartar:** Hard deposit on the teeth near the gum line formed by plaque build-up and dead bacteria.
- **Thrill:** Palpable feeling caused by turbulent blood flow.
- **Thrombophlebitis:** A blood clot that accompanies vein inflammation.
- **Thrombosis:** The formation or development of a blood clot.
- **Tracheostomy:** Curved tube inserted into an artificial opening made into the trachea; comes in varied angles and multiple sizes.
- **Trans fat:** Product that results when liquid oils are partially hydrogenated; these oils then become more stable and solid; trans fats raise serum cholesterol levels.
- **Transmission-based precautions:** Precautions used in addition to Standard Precautions for patients in hospitals who are suspected of being infected with pathogens that can be transmitted by airborne, droplet, or contact routes; these precautions encompass all the diseases or conditions previously listed in the disease specific or category-specific classifications.

- **Triglycerides:** Predominant form of fat in food and the major storage form of fat in the body; composed of one glyceride molecule and three fatty acids.
- **Tunneling:** Passageway or opening that may be visible at skin level, but with most of the tunnel under the surface of the skin.
- **Typing:** Determining a person's blood type (A, B, AB, or O).
- **Undermining:** Areas of tissue destruction underneath intact skin along the margins of a wound; associated with Stage 3 or 4 pressure ulcers.
- **Vagal stimulus or response:** Stimulation of the vagus nerve that causes an increase in parasympathetic stimulation, triggering a decrease in heart rate.
- **Valsalva maneuver:** Voluntary contraction of the abdominal wall muscles, fixing of the diaphragm, and closing of the glottis that increases intra-abdominal pressure and aids in expelling feces.
- **Vasoconstriction:** Narrowing of the lumen of a blood vessel.
- **Vasodilation:** An increase in the diameter of a blood vessel.
- **Venous stasis:** Decrease in blood flow in the venous system related to dysfunctional valves or inactivity of the muscles of the affected extremity.
- Ventilation (breathing): The movement of air into and out of the lungs.
- **Vial:** A glass bottle with a self-sealing stopper through which medication is removed.
- **Vitamins:** Organic substances needed by the body in small amounts to help regulate body processes; are susceptible to oxidation and destruction.

NURSING PROCESS

DEFINITION

A nursing process is a tool or method for organizing and delivering care or a deliberate intellectual activity whereby the practice of nursing is approached in an orderly systematic manner. It is a systematic problem-solving approach to client care. It is a series of planned steps and actions directed toward meeting the need and solving the problems of people and their significant others; it is systematic, scientific problem-solving in action.

PURPOSES OF NURSING PROCESS

- To identify the client's health care needs.
- To establish nursing care plan so as to meet those needs.
- To complete the nursing intervention designed to meet the needs.
- To provide individualized care.

STEPS OF THE NURSING PROCESS

The nursing process has five steps:

1. Assessment

Assessment is the systematic collection of data to determine the patient's health status and to identify any actual or potential health problems. In nursing assessment, the best sources of information about the client are the client and the family. Health professionals, previous client records and significant others also act as information sources. Data collected about a client generally fall into one of the two categories: objective or subjective.

Objective data: It includes all the measurable and observable pieces of information about the client and his or her overall state of health. The term objective means that only precise, accurate measurements or clear descriptions are used.

Subjective data: It consists the client's opinions and feelings about what is happening. Only the client can tell you that he/she is afraid or has pain. Sometimes the client can communicate through body language: gesture, facial expressions and body posture. To obtain subjective data you need sharp interviewing, listening, and observation skills.

Methods of data collection:

Observation is an assessment tool that relies on the use of five senses (sight, touch, hearing, smell, and taste) to discover information about the client.

Health interview is a way of soliciting information from the client. This interview may also be called a nursing history.

2. Diagnosis

Nursing diagnosis: Actual or potential health problems that can be managed by independent nursing interventions.

Purposes of the nursing diagnosis:

- Identifies nursing priorities.
- Directs nursing interventions to meet the client's high priority needs.
- Provides a common language and forms a basis for communication and understanding between nursing professionals and health care team.

- Guides the formulation of expected outcomes for quality assurance requirements of third-party payer.
- Provides a basis for evaluation to determine if nursing care was beneficial to the client and cost effective.

The diagnostic statement:

The client may present with more than one problem. Therefore, the nursing diagnosis may be made up of multiple *diagnostic statements*. Each diagnostic statement has two or three parts depending on the healthcare facility. The three-part statement consists of the following components:

- Problem
- Etiology
- Signs and symptoms

And a two-part diagnostic statement consists of the problem, and signs and symptoms.

Problem: The problem portion of a statement describes the health problem of a client clearly and concisely. Use one of the NANDA Approved nursing diagnostic labels to state the problem.

Etiology: The Etiology part of the diagnostic statement is the cause of the problem. Etiology may be physiological, psychological, sociological, spiritual, or environmental.

Signs and symptoms: The third part of the diagnostic statement summarizes data. You may need to include several signs and symptoms. For instance, the client with pneumonia had cough with thick sputum, abnormal breath sounds, increased respiration, and difficulty breathing.

Writing the diagnostic statement:

The diagnostic statement connects problem, etiology, and signs and symptoms. The first two parts of the statement are linked by "related to", sometimes abbreviated R/T. The last two parts are linked by "as evidenced by", sometimes abbreviated AEB.

For example, Ineffective Airway Clearance related to physiologic effects of pneumonia as evidenced by increased sputum, coughing, abnormal breath sounds, tachypnea, and dyspnea.

Collaborative Problems are certain physiologic complications that nurse monitors to detect onset or changes in status. Nurses manage collaborative problems using physician-prescribed and nursing-prescribed interventions to minimize the complications of the events.

3. Planning

The development of goals and a plan of care designed to assist the patient in resolving the diagnosed problems. Setting priorities, establishing expected outcomes, and selecting nursing interventions result in plan of nursing care.

Setting priorities:

Nursing diagnoses are ranked in order of importance. Survival needs or imminent life-threatening situations take the highest priority. For example, the needs for air, water and food are survival needs. Nursing diagnostic categories that reflect these high priority needs include Ineffective Airway Clearance and deficient fluid volume.

Establishing expected outcomes:

An expected outcome is a measurable client behavior that indicates whether the person has achieved the expected benefit of nursing care. It may also be called a *goal* or *objective.* An expected outcome has the following characteristics:

- Client-oriented
- Specific
- Reasonable
- Measurable.

Selecting nursing interventions:

Nursing intervention is also called nursing orders or nursing actions, are activities that will most likely produce the desired outcomes (short-term or long-term). To achieve this outcome, one should select nursing interventions such as the following examples:

- Offering fluids frequently
- Positioning frequently
- Teaching deep breathing exercises
- Monitoring vital signs
- Administering oxygen, etc. accordingly.

4. Implementation

Actualization of the plan of care through nursing interventions.

5. Evaluation

Determination of the patient's responses to the nursing intervention and the extent to which the goals have been achieved.

HEALTH ASSESSMENT

Health: A state of complete physical, mental and social well-being and not merely the absence of disease or infirmity.

—**WHO 1998**

Assessment: "Assessment is a systematic, dynamic process by which the nurse through interaction with client, significant others and health care providers, collects and analyzes data about client." —**American Nurses Association**

Health Assessment is a regular and conscious process. This is an important tool to determine the health status of an individual. It consists of a systematic and orderly collection of information pertaining to the health status of the client. Assessment includes subjective data through interviewing the client and obtaining objective data by physically examining the client. Subjective data are those symptoms, values and information that only the client can state and validate. Objective data can be directly measured and observed such as vital signs or patient of the patient.

Purposes of the Health Assessment

- To establish the data for the client's normal abilities, risk factors or any current alteration in function.
- To plan strategies to encourage the continuation of the healthy pattern, prevent potential health problems and alleviate or manage existing health problems.
- To provide a holistic view of the client.
- To provide an essential foundation for the care of the client.
- To develop (obtain baseline data) and expand the database from which subsequent phases of the nursing process can evolve.
- To identify and manage a variety of patient problems (actual and potential).
- To supplement, confirm, or refute data obtained in the nursing history.
- To obtain data that will help establish nursing diagnoses and nursing plans of care.
- To evaluate the physiological outcomes of health care and thus the progress of a client's health problem.
- To make clinical judgments about a client's health status.
- To identify areas for health promotion and disease prevention.

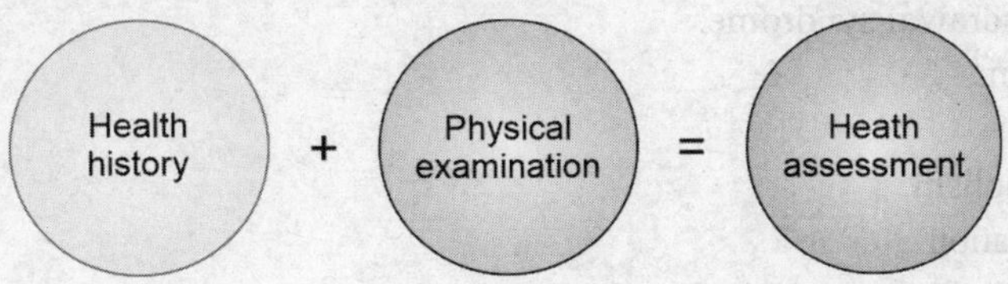

Health History

Health history is a collection of subjective data that includes information on both the client's past and present health status.

Following are the components of the history taking:

- Biodemographic data of patient
- Patient complaints
- History of present illness
- Past media history
- Medical history
- Medication history
- Socioeconomic status
- Family history of any illness
- Developmental history
- Menstrual history
- Obstetrical history

- Family history
- Functional health pattern
- Environmental history
- Physical examination.
- Blood pathological investigation
- Radiodiagnostic investigation
- Medication
- Patient feedback
- Summary
- Reference

NANDA—NURSING DIAGNOSIS

A nursing diagnosis is defined by NANDA International as a clinical judgment concerning a human response to health conditions/life processes, or vulnerability for that response, by an individual, family, group, or community.

New NANDA nursing diagnoses:

- Readiness for enhanced health literacy
- Ineffective adolescent eating dynamics
- Ineffective child eating dynamics
- Ineffective infant eating dynamics
- Risk for metabolic imbalance syndrome
- Imbalanced energy field
- Risk for unstable blood pressure
- Risk for complicated immigration transition
- Neonatal abstinence syndrome
- Acute substance withdrawal syndrome.
- Risk for acute substance withdrawal syndrome.
- Risk for surgical site infection.
- Risk for dry mouth.
- Risk for venous thromboembolism.
- Risk for female genital mutilation.
- Risk for occupational injury.
- Risk for ineffective thermoregulation

INFECTION CONTROL IN CLINICAL SETTINGS

INTRODUCTION

Nurses are involved in providing a biologically safe environment and promoting health. Microorganisms exist everywhere in the environment; in water, soil and body surfaces such as skin, intestinal tract, and other areas open to the outside.

Infection is the process of bacteria or viruses invading the body or making someone ill or diseased. When you catch a cold, this is an example of an infection. A virus is an example of an infection.

Infection control is the discipline concerned with preventing nosocomial or healthcare-associated infection. It is an essential (though often under-recognized and under-supported) part of the infrastructure of health care.

NATURE OF INFECTION

- Microorganisms: bacteria, fungi, viruses, protozoa and worms
- Most are harmless (non-pathogenic)
- Pathogenic organisms can cause infection
- Infection exists when pathogenic organisms enter the body, reproduce and cause disease

CHAIN OF INFECTION

There are six links in the chain of infection:

1. The etiologic agent, or microorganism:
2. The reservoir, the place where the organism naturally resides.
3. Portal of exit from reservoir
4. Method of transmission
5. Portal of entry into the host
6. Susceptibility of the host.

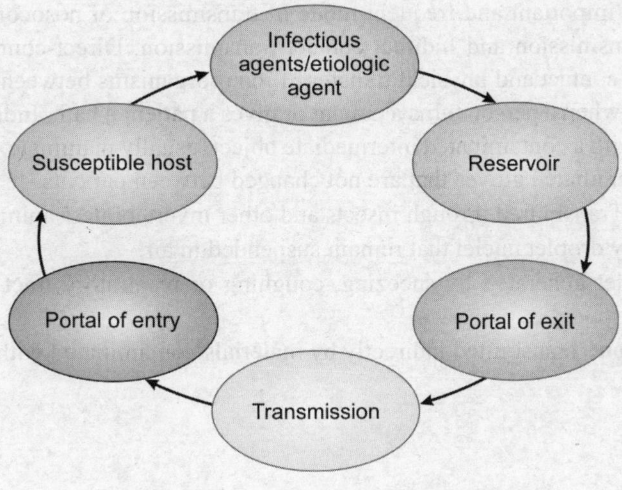

TYPES OF INFECTION

- **Primary infection**
  - Initial infection with an organism to host constitutes primary infection.

- **Secondary infection**
  - When a host's resistance is lowered by pre-existing infection, a new organism may set up a new infection.

STAGES OF INFECTION

- **Incubation period:** Time from initial contact to first signs of symptoms.
- **Prodrome period:** 1–2 days of initial symptoms.
- **Invasion period:** Multiplies at high levels, reached target tissue, greatest toxicity during this stage.
- **Convalescent period:** Recovery period.

NOSOCOMIAL INFECTION

Hospital acquired infections are considered nosocomial if they first appear 48 hours or more after hospital admission or within 30 days after discharge. There is rise in nosocomial infection as a result of four factors:

- Crowded hospital conditions
- New microorganisms
- Increased number of people with compromised immune system
- Increased bacterial resistance

EPIDEMIOLOGY

Nosocomial infections can be exogenous (external organism) and endogenous (opportunist normal flora). Host susceptibility is an important factor in the development of nosocomial infections. Medical equipment and procedures (surgery) are often responsible for infections.

MODES OF TRANSMISSION

There are five main modes of transmission: Contact, Vector borne, Air borne, Droplet, Common vehicle.

1. **Contact transmission:** Most important and frequent mode of transmission of nosocomial infections is divided into two subgroups: Direct-contact transmission and Indirect-contact transmission. Direct-contact transmission involves a direct body surface-to-body surface contact and physical transfer of microorganisms between a susceptible host and an infected or colonized person. It occurs when a person turns a patient or gives a patient a bath. Indirect-contact transmission involves contact of a susceptible host with a contaminated intermediate object, usually inanimate, such as contaminated instruments, needles, or dressings, or contaminated gloves that are not changed between patients.
2. **Vector borne transmission:** Transmitted through insects and other invertebrates' animals such as mosquitoes and fleas.
3. **Air borne transmission:** Tiny droplet nuclei that remain suspended in air.
4. **Droplet transmission:** Droplet generated by sneezing, coughing or respiratory tract procedures like bronchoscopy or suction.
5. **Common vehicle transmission:** Transmitted indirectly by materials contaminated with the infections.

COMMON INFECTIONS

Following are the most common nosocomial infections: Urinary tract infection, catheter associated infection, pneumonia, blood stream infections.

PROBLEMS OF NOSOCOMIAL INFECTIONS

Nosocomial infections will become more important like public health problems as they cause nosocomial suffering and thus prolonged hospital stay increases the cost of care significantly.

- **Surgical site infections:** They are frequent as the infection is mainly clinical (purulent discharge around wounds or the insertion site of drain, or spreading cellulites from wounds). The infections can be exogenous or endogenous.
- **Nosocomial pneumonia:** The most important are patients on ventilators in ICU. Recent and progressive radiological opacities of the pulmonary parenchyma, purulent sputum and recent onsite fever. Most common are caused by acinetobacter.
- **Nosocomial bacteremia:** The incidence is increasing particularly for certain organisms such as multi resistance coagulate negative staphylococcus and candida. Infections may occur at the skin entry site of the IV device or in the subcutaneous path of catheter.
- **Urinary tract infection:** It is the most common cause of nosocomial infections. 80% of the infections are associated with indwelling catheters.

PREVENTION AND CONTROL

Prevention and control of nosocomial infections can be done by the following ways. Isolation is designed to prevent transmission of microorganisms by common routes in hospitals. Because agent and host factors are more difficult to control, interruption of transfer of microorganisms is directed primarily at transmission.

- Sterilization of all reusable equipment such as ventilator, humidifier and any device that come in contact with the respiratory tract.
- Wear gloves for two reasons, they provide a protective barrier and prevent contamination of hands and reduce the likelihood that microorganisms present on the hands will be transmitted to the patients during invasive and other patient care procedures.
- Wear aprons as during patient care, an apron reduces the risk of infections. Apron is must for preventing yourself from catching infection.
- Get educated about your conditions and treatment is the best way to prevent an error. Get involved and be assertive about your rights to be a part of the decision process for your medical care.

HAND HYGIENE

Hand hygiene: It refers to the practices used to prevent and control the spread of pathogenic organisms. It protects the patient and his/her environment from the transmission of disease producing organisms.

Purposes:

- For aesthetic sense
- To cleans the hands
- To minimize microbial content of the hands
- To prevent cross infection from patients, to self and vice versa

Steps of hand hygiene:

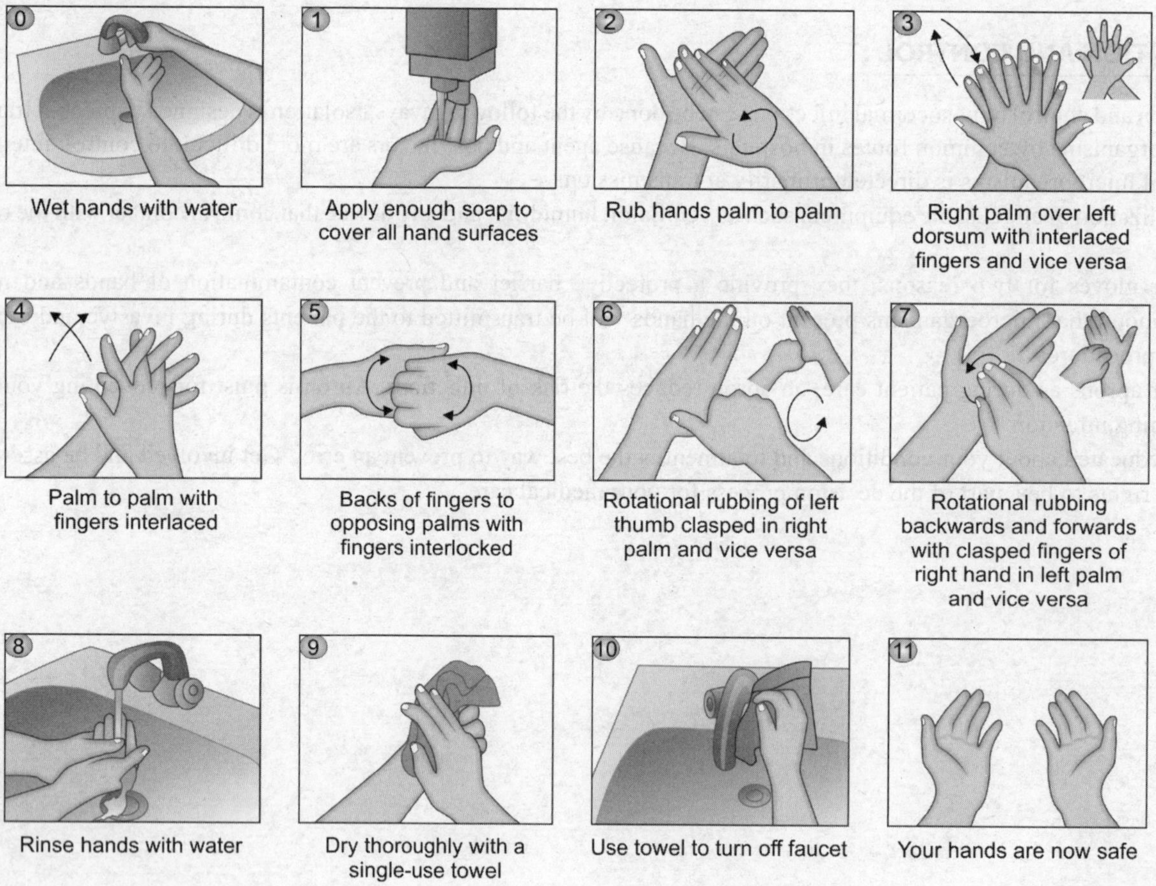

Moments of Hand Washing:

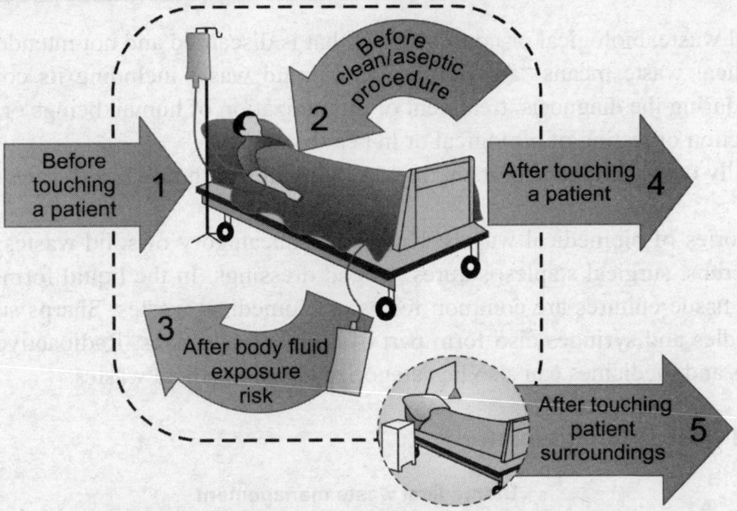

1	Before touching a patient	**When?** Clean your hands before touching a patient when approaching him/her. **Why?** To protect the patient against harmful germs carried on your hands.
2	Before clean/aseptic procedure	**When?** Clean your hands immediately before performing a clean/aseptic procedure. **Why?** To protect the patient against harmful germs, including the patient's own entering his/her body.
3	After body fluid exposure risk	**When?** Clean your hands immediately after an exposure risk to body fluids (and after glove removal). **Why?** To protect yourself and the health-care environment from harmful patient germs.
4	Afer touching a patient	**When?** Clean your hands after touching a patient and her/his immediate surroundings, when leaving the patient's side. **Why?** To protect yourself and the health-care environment from harmful patient germs.
5	After touching patient surroundings	**When?** Clean your hands after touching any object or furniture in the patient's immediate surroundings, when leaving—even if the patient has not been touched. **Why?** To protect yourself and the health-care environment from harmful patient germs.

BIOMEDICAL HOSPITAL WASTE MANAGEMENT

Hospital waste: Refers to all waste, biological or nonbiological that is discarded and not intended for further use.

Biomedical waste: Biomedical waste means "any solid and/or liquid waste including its container and any intermediate product, which is generated during the diagnosis, treatment or immunization of human beings or animals or research activities pertaining to or in the production or testing of biological or in health camps."

Biomedical wastes usually occur in clinics, nursing homes, laboratories, home health care, veterinarian clinics and other similar places.

There are various categories of biomedical wastes. Under the subcategory of solid wastes, there come catheters, tubes, disposable gowns, masks, scrubs, surgical staples, sutures, wound dressings. In the liquid forms of biomedical wastes, body fluids, tissues, cells, organs, tissue cultures are common forms of biomedical wastes. Sharps such as blades, razors, scalpel, lancets, cuvettes, slides, needles and syringes also form part of biomedical wastes. Radioactive materials, different types of pharmacological concoctions and medicines can also be categorized as biomedical wastes.

Categories of Biomedical Waste Management

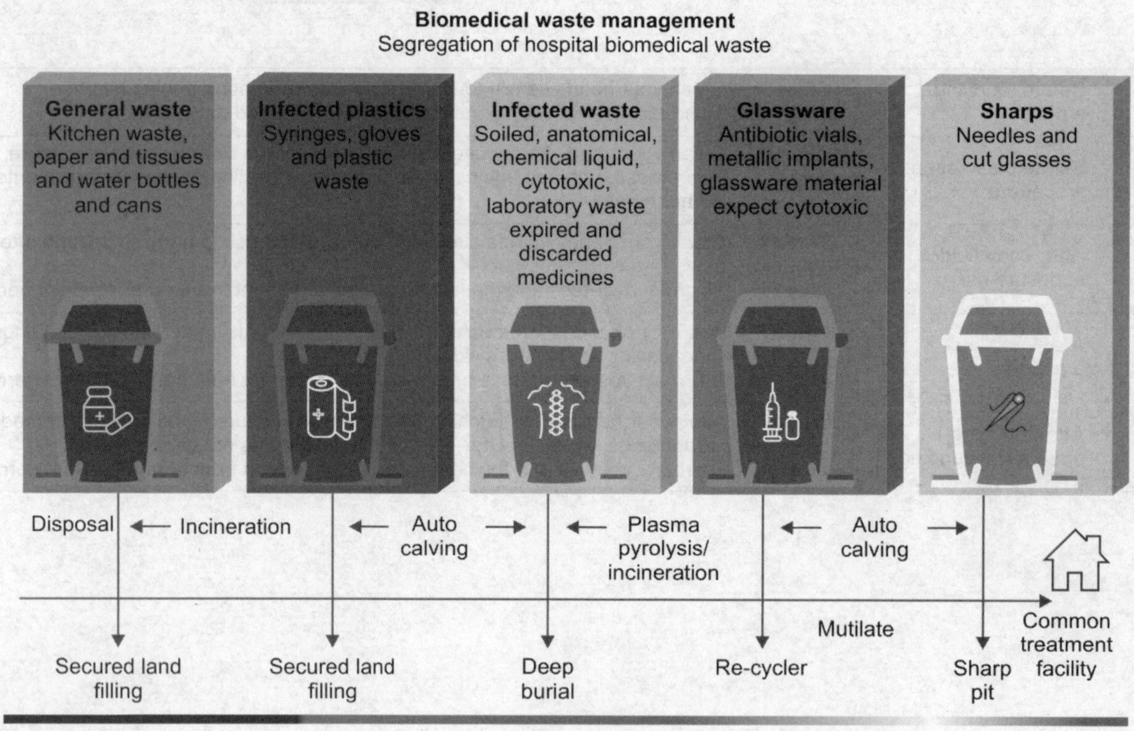

PERSONAL PROTECTIVE EQUIPMENT (PPE)

How to put on PPE (when all PPE items are needed)

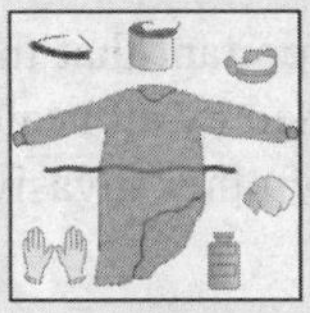

Step 1
- Identify hazards and manage risk. Gather the necessary PPE.
- Plan where to put on and take of PPE.
- Do you have a buddy? Mirror?
- Do you know how you will deal with waste?

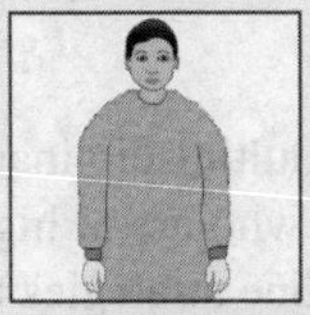

Step 2
- Put on a gown.

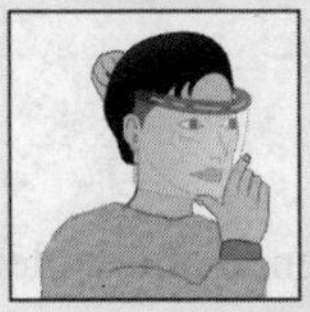

Step 3a
- Put on face shield.

or

Step 3b
- Put on medical mask and eye protection (e.g. eye visor/goggles).

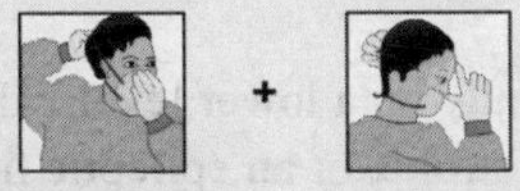

Note: If performing an aerosol-generating procedure (e.g. aspiration of respiratory tract, intubation, resuscitation, bronchoscopy, autopsy), a particulate respirator (e.g. US NIOSH-certified N95, EU FFP2, or equivalent respirator) should be used in combination with a face shield or an eye protection. Do user seal check if using a particulate respirator.

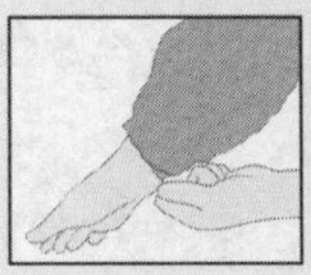

Step 4
- Put on gloves (over cuff).

How to take off PPE

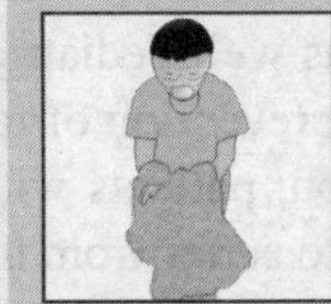

Step 1
- Avoid contamination of self, others and the environment.
- Remove the most heavily contaminated items first.

Remove gloves and gown
- Peel off gown and gloves and roll inside, out.
- Dispose gloves and gown safely.

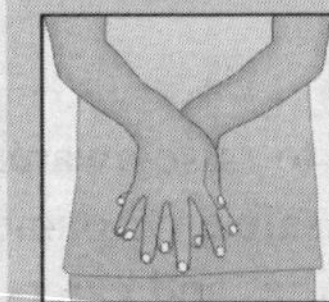

Step 2
- Perform hand hygiene.

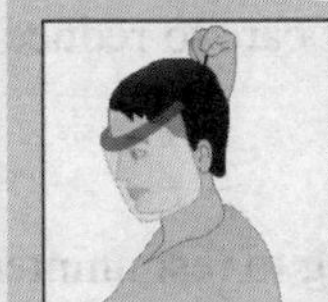

Step 3a
If wearing face shield:
- Remove face shield from behind.
- Dispose of face shield safely.

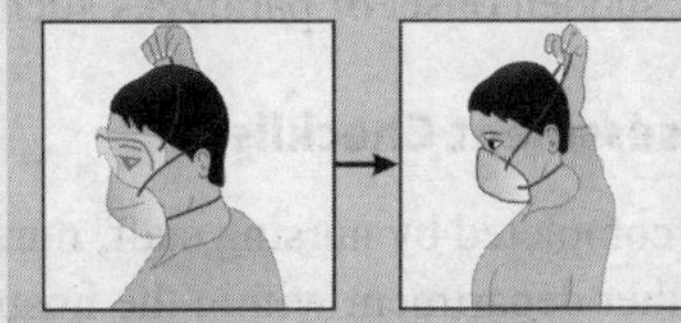

Step 3b
If wearing eye protection and mask:
- Remove goggles from behind.
- Put goggles in a separate container for reprocessing.
- Remove mask from behind and dispose of safely.

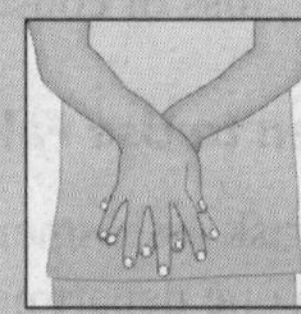

Step 4
- Perform hand hygiene.

According to the World Health Organization (WHO), personal protective equipment "consists of garments placed to protect the health care workers or any other persons to get infected."

FALL RISK ASSESSMENT

Introduction

Falls are the most common cause of adult as well pediatric injury during the hospitalization period. It is important that this close observation and monitoring about the prevention of falls in the hospital environment need to be performed by all health care professionals. During the hospitalization, patients with mechanical ventilators or those who are on any other invasive equipment and elder people are more prone to suffer from the fall risk.

Aim

The intention of this fall risk assessment is, to raise awareness and educate nursing staff, students, and the multidisciplinary team about the importance of maintaining a safe environment for all patients; assist with identifying patients who are at high risk of fall; provide the tools to educate families and carers of the patients with potential risk of falls and outline strategies to develop individualized management plans of care to reduce the risk for high-risk patients.

Definition

Fall: Fall is an event, which results in coming to rest unintentionally on a lower level, other than as a consequence of a violent blow, loss of consciousness, sudden onset of paralyzes such as a stroke, or an epileptic fit during the hospitalization.

When to Use Fall Risk Assessment Checklist

Fall risk assessment is to be completed by nursing staff, nursing students and nurses in the hospital on admission, after transfer from one department to another department within the hospital, two weeks after admission, after an acute episode or fall, and after the post-operative or critical condition at critical care unit every two hourly.

Falls Risk Factors

Age: Falls mostly occur in elderly people and children during the hospitalization period.

Falls history: History of falling is the information that can be obtained from the incident reports and patient's history.

Mobility/activity and balance: If the resident is immobile or bed-bound and not likely to improve this question is not applicable and you should tick "No".

If the patient is mobile and gaiting or is restrained for the prevention of activities, the patient should be closely monitored or fall risk prevention action should be taken.

Mental state: Patients with disturbed mental status and affected with the mental disorders are more prone to risk of fall in the hospitals.

Sensory: Bed-ridden and immobile patients need to be monitored for the sensory function of the patients during the care on a regular basis. Sensory function loss may be found in stroke, bed-ridden patients, patients with sedation and may be prone to the fall risk.

Medications

- Antihypertensive
- Vasodilators
- Diuretics
- Antiparkinsonians
- Vestibular depressants

Medications

Number of medications: This refers to any medications taken, prescription and non-prescription, irrespective of its medication category (specific medication categories are covered in the question related to "type of medication" taken–see below).

Those medications are associated with an increased risk for falls. For example, antipsychotic, sedatives, etc. are need to be monitored for medication dose and route and their adverse effects if any.

Transfers and Gait

If the patient is immobile or bed-bound and not likely to improve, this question is not applicable and you should tick "No". Otherwise, record transfer and mobility status using the listed options.